Varus Ankle, Foot, and Tibia

Guest Editor

ALASTAIR S. YOUNGER, MD, ChB, FRCSC

FOOT AND ANKLE CLINICS

www.foot.theclinics.com

Consulting Editor
MARK S. MYERSON, MD

March 2012 • Volume 17 • Number 1

SAUNDERS an imprint of ELSEVIER, Inc.

W.B. SAUNDERS COMPANY
A Division of Elsevier Inc.

1600 John F. Kennedy Blvd. • Suite 1800 • Philadelphia, PA 19103-2899

http://www.theclinics.com

FOOT AND ANKLE CLINICS Volume 17, Number 1
March 2012 ISSN 1083-7515, ISBN-13: 978-1-4557-3861-8

Editor: David Parsons

Foot and Ankle Clinics (ISSN 1083-7515) is published quarterly by Elsevier, Inc., 360 Park Avenue South, New York, NY 10010-1710. Months of issue are March, June, September, and December. Periodicals postage paid at New York, NY, and additional mailing offices. Subscription price per year is $295.00 (US individuals), $386.00 (US institutions), $146.00 (US students), $336.00 (Canadian individuals), $456.00 (Canadian institutions), $201.00 (Canadian students), $433.00 (foreign individuals), $456.00 (foreign institutions), and $201.00 (foreign students). To receive student/resident rate, orders must be accompanied by name of affiliated institution, date of term, and the signature of program/residency coordinator on institution letterhead. Orders will be billed at individual rate until proof of status is received. Foreign air speed delivery is included in all *Clinics* subscription prices. All prices are subject to change without notice. **POSTMASTER:** Send address changes to *Foot and Ankle Clinics,* Elsevier Health Sciences Division, Subscription Customer Service, 3251 Riverport Lane, Maryland Heights, MO 63043. **Customer Service: 1-800-654-2452 (US and Canada). From outside of the United States and Canada, call 314-447-8871. Fax: 314-447-8029. E-mail: JournalsCustomerService-usa@elsevier.com (for print support); JournalsOnlineSupport-usa@elsevier.com (for online support).**

Reprints. For copies of 100 or more, of articles in this publication, please contact the Commercial Reprints Department, Elsevier Inc., 360 Park Avenue South, New York, NY 10010-1710. Tel.: 212-633-3812; Fax: 212-462-1935; E-mail: reprints@elsevier.com.

Printed and bound by CPI Group (UK) Ltd, Croydon, CR0 4YY

Transferred to Digital Print 2012

Contributors

CONSULTING EDITOR

MARK S. MYERSON, MD
Director, Institute for Foot and Ankle Reconstruction at Mercy, Mercy Medical Center, Baltimore, Maryland

GUEST EDITOR

ALASTAIR S. YOUNGER, MD, ChB, FRCSC
Associate Professor, Department of Orthopaedics, University of British Columbia, British Columbia's Foot and Ankle Clinic, St. Pauls Hospital, Vancouver, British Columbia, Canada

AUTHORS

KELLY L. APOSTLE, MD, FRCSC
Fellow, Harborview Medical Center, Seattle, Washington

DOUGLAS BEAMAN, MD
Summit Orthopedic, Portland, Oregon

EMANUEL BENNINGER, MD
Consultant, Foot and Ankle Surgery, Department of Orthopaedics, University of Zurich, Balgrist, Zurich, Switzerland

LILIANNA BOLLIGER, MSc
Department of Orthopaedic Surgery, Kantonsspital Liestal, Liestal, Switzerland

TIMOTHY R. DANIELS, MD, FRCS(C)
Associate Professor, Head of Foot & Ankle Program, University of Toronto; Staff Surgeon, St. Michael's Hospital, Toronto, Ontario, Canada

MARK E. EASLEY, MD
Associate Professor and co-director of the Foot & Ankle Fellowship, Department of Orthopaedics, Duke University, Durham, North Carolina

NORMAN ESPINOSA, MD
Head of Foot and Ankle Surgery, Department of Orthopaedics, University of Zurich, Balgrist, Zurich, Switzerland

RICHARD GELLMAN, MD
Summit Orthopedic, Portland, Oregon

MARK A. GLAZEBROOK, MD, MSc, PhD, FRCSC
Associate Professor, Department of Orthopaedic Surgery, QEII Health Sciences Centre, Halifax Infirmary, Halifax, Nova Scotia, Canada

BEAT HINTERMANN, MD
Department of Orthopaedic Surgery, Kantonsspital Liestal, Liestal, Switzerland

LUKAS D. ISELIN, MD
Royal Adelaide Hospital, Orthopaedic and Trauma Service, North Terrace, Adelaide,
South Australia, Australia

GEORG KLAMMER, MD
Consultant, Foot and Ankle Surgery, Department of Orthopaedics, University of Zurich,
Balgrist, Zurich, Switzerland

MARKUS KNUPP, MD
Department of Orthopaedic Surgery, Kantonsspital Liestal, Liestal, Switzerland

FABIAN G. KRAUSE, MD
Department of Orthopaedic Surgery, Inselspital, University of Bern, Bern, Switzerland

D. JOSH MAYICH, MD, FRCS(C)
St. Michael's Hospital, Toronto, Ontario, Canada

MARK S. MYERSON, MD
Director, Institute for Foot and Ankle Reconstruction at Mercy, Mercy Medical Center,
Baltimore, Maryland

BRUCE J. SANGEORZAN, MD
Veterans Administration Center of Excellence for Limb Loss Prevention and Prosthetic
Engineering; University of Washington; Department of Orthopaedics and Sports
Medicine, Harborview Medical Center, Seattle, Washington

JAMES A. SPROULE, MB, BAO, BCh, MCh, FRCSI, FRCS (Tr & Orth)
Clinical Fellow, Department of Orthopaedic Surgery, QEII Health Sciences Centre,
Halifax Infirmary, Halifax, Nova Scotia, Canada

KEN-JIN TAN, MBBS, MRCS, FRCS
Associate Consultant, Division of Foot and Ankle Surgery, University Orthopaedics
Hand and Reconstructive Microsurgery Cluster, National University Hospital, Singapore

GOWREESON THEVENDRAN, FRCS (Tr & Ortho)
Fellow in Foot and Ankle Surgery, St. Paul's Hospital, Vancouver, British Columbia,
Canada

J. CARR VINEYARD, MD
W.B. Carrell Memorial Clinic, Dallas, Texas

ALASTAIR S. YOUNGER, MD, ChB, FRCSC
Associate Professor, Department of Orthopaedics, University of British Columbia, British
Columbia's Foot and Ankle Clinic, St. Pauls Hospital, Vancouver, British Columbia, Canada

Contents

> Varus deformity of the foot and ankle encompasses a spectrum of conditions from mild to severe. The cause of this deformity may be bone, muscle imbalance, or a combination of both. An understanding of the anatomic variations seen in each individual patient is essential for planning surgical intervention. The authors outline the anatomic variations that cause and are a consequence of varus deformities of the foot and ankle.

> Varus malalignment of the distal lower extremity can be challenging to treat. There can be a spectrum of involvement of the cavus foot. The varus hindfoot may result in lateral ankle instability with continuous attenuation of the lateral collateral ligaments. The varus tibia may be secondary to a variety of causes. Ultimately, physical examination supersedes all other investigations. After investigations have been performed, the patient needs to be reviewed and the results interpreted in light of the clinical findings. At this point the examiner will be able to determine what is significant and decide on an appropriate treatment plan.

> To our knowledge, little is reported about the management of the patients with combined symptomatic osteochondral lesions of the talus (OLT) and varus ankle malalignment. Treatment strategies for symptomatic OLTs are relatively well-described in the orthopedic literature. Although less defined than the surgical management of OLTs, realignment procedures for the varus ankle and hindfoot have also been studied and reported in some detail, albeit with a focus on management of ankle arthritis. In this article, we review practical concepts from the orthopedic literature that may be applied when treating patients with concomitant OLTs and varus ankles malalignment.

> Muscle imbalance from underlying neurologic disorders can cause hindfoot varus deformity. Most etiologies are congenital, and therefore affect bone morphology and the shape of the foot during growth. Treatment decisions in varus hindfoot caused by neurologic disorders must be individualized. Deformity corrections include release of soft tissue contractures, osteotomies and arthrodeses, and tenotomies or tendon transfers to balance muscle strength and prevent recurrence. The goal of static and dynamic hindfoot varus realignment is to fully correct all components of the deformity, but particularly the varus tilt of the talus.

> Varus ankle associated with instability can be simple or complex. Multiple underlying diseases may contribute to this complex pathologic entity. These conditions should be recognized when attempting proper decision-making. Treatment options range from conservative measures to surgical reconstruction. Whereas conservative treatment might be a possible approach for patients with simple varus ankle instability, more complex instabilities require extensive surgical reconstructions. However, adequate diagnostic workup and accurate analysis of varus ankle instability provide a base for the successful treatment outcome.

> We recommend gradual correction of distal tibial varus as most applicable in patients with severe deformities who would not be adequately corrected with acute methods. Complex deformity, compromised soft tissues, and limb shortening are, in general, better managed with this technique.

> A majority of patients with posttraumatic arthritis of the ankle joint present with a malaligned hindfoot. Young patients with midstage arthritis have been shown to benefit from alignment surgery with regard to the functional, subjective, and radiologic outcome. However, due to the complex build of the ankle joint, normalization of intraarticular load distribution may require not only correction of the distal tibial articular surface angle but also additional procedures such as sagittal plane correction and adjustment of the fibular length and orientation.

Ankle replacement in the presence of a varus deformity is an evolving field. Although initial results were disappointing, numerous advances in the understanding of the condition and surgical techniques have been made. More recent reports show good short-term results, especially when adjunctive procedures are combined to achieve a neutral alignment and restore lateral ligamentous stability. It is possible to correct varus deformities of 20° or more with ankle replacement. It is likely with a reliable correction of alignment and balance that the long-term results of ankle replacement in significant varus deformity will be promising.

The architectural integrity of the talus is instrumental in assuring normal foot function. Posttraumatic malalignment after talar neck fracture inevitably predisposes to painful functional impairment. Treatment of talar neck malunion is difficult. Prevention through accurate reduction and definitive, stable osteosynthesis at primary surgery is important. In the absence of arthrosis in the peritalar articulations, delayed anatomic reconstruction can be considered. Although a plantigrade foot can be achieved with reorientating arthrodeses, functional impairment prevails, and the long-term outcome is compromised because of the development of degenerative changes in the adjacent joints.

Varus malalignment of the ankle (VMAA) is a misleading term. The isolated frontal plane deformity is multiplanar. Identifying this dominant feature and applying appropriate surgical principles to allow for complete correction of the deformity are important for a successful surgical outcome. Three factors are key to optimal outcomes from total ankle replacements (TAR): (1) Obtaining a congruent ankle with sufficient ROM is necessary before implantation of the prosthesis; (2) not all varus ankles are correctable; and (3) recognition both preoperatively and intraoperatively that conversion of TAR to fusion is sometimes the best way to achieve optimal results for the patient. Varus malalignment of the ankle (VMAA) measuring greater than 10° is a technical challenge for any surgeon performing total ankle replacements (TAR). The current literature is composed of mostly level III and V evidence and does not provide the surgeon with a reliable treatment algorithm.

THE CLINICS ARE NOW AVAILABLE ONLINE!

Access your subscription at:
www.theclinics.com

Preface
Cavus Foot

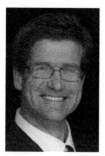

Alastair S. Younger, MD, ChB, FRCSC
Guest Editor

I would like to say thank you to everybody involved in this edition. First, I would like to thank Mark Myerson for inviting me to do this edition. Mark should be recognized also for his tireless devotion to *Foot and Ankle Clinics*. To keep working away the way he does getting these high-quality articles out year after year deserves special mention.

I would also like to thank all the authors. These were very high-quality articles that required little editing and I learned a lot by reading them. I hope you as a reader of this edition enjoy and learn from them as I did. As a result, my job as guest editor was very easy.

This was truly an international group, and I would like to thank all of our non–North American authors, who did a spectacular job producing articles in English. Like many English speakers, I am completely unilingual and would not be able to begin to translate my article into acceptable French or German. For the fact that I don't have to translate, I am grateful.

I would also like to thank the staff at Elsevier and David Parsons in particular for doing the real work of getting this edition out. I would also like to thank them for their continued dedication to foot and ankle education.

So read on and enjoy!

Alastair S. Younger, MD, ChB, FRCSC
Department of Orthopaedics
University of British Columbia
British Columbia's Foot and Ankle Clinic
St. Pauls Hospital
560 1144 Burrard Street
Vancouver, BC V6Z 2A5, Canada

E-mail address:
asyounger@telus.net

Foot Ankle Clin N Am 17 (2012) ix
doi:10.1016/j.fcl.2011.11.010
1083-7515/12/$ – see front matter

Anatomy of the Varus Foot and Ankle

Kelly L. Apostle, MD, FRCSC[a],*, Bruce J. Sangeorzan, MD[b,c,d]

KEYWORDS
- Foot and ankle • Anatomy • Varus deformity
- Foot biomechanics

Varus deformity implies angulation toward the midline of the distal segment of bone or joint. Because the foot is at a right angle to the long axis of the leg, use of the term in the foot may be confusing. Varus of the ankle refers to a varus plafond or varus tilt of the talus in the mortise. Varus of the hindfoot refers to angulation toward the midline of the longitudinal axis of the calcaneal tuberosity and may also be referred to as supination, or inversion of the subtalar joint. Varus of the forefoot refers to elevation of the medial ray and may also be referred to as supination or inversion of the plane of the metatarsal heads relative to the hindfoot (**Fig. 1**). Varus deformity of the foot and ankle is common and embodies a spectrum of anatomic variations from mild to severe, and in many cases is completely asymptomatic. Varus of the foot and ankle is often associated with a pes cavus deformity but may also occur with a low or normal arch.

The cause of the varus deformity may be bone, muscle imbalance, or a combination of both. Common osseous abnormalities leading to varus of the ankle and foot include varus malunion of the tibial plafond, talus and calcaneus, residual clubfoot, and tarsal coalition. Muscle imbalance may be caused by hereditary motor sensory neuropathies, cerebral palsy, stroke, sequelae of compartment syndrome, nerve injury, or primary spinal pathology. Alternatively, patients may present with no clear underlying cause; however, a careful assessment of the patient's anatomy is likely to reveal subtle variations from normal contributing to the clinical condition. Initially, many of these pathologic conditions begin as compensable deformities. Over time they may become rigid, leading to anatomic abnormalities that in turn impart

Funding: No funding was received for the current article.
Disclosure: KL Apostle: nothing to disclose. BJ Sangeorzan: nothing to disclose.
[a] Harborview Medical Center, 325 Ninth Avenue, Seattle, WA 98104, USA
[b] Veterans Administration Center of Excellence for Limb Loss Prevention and Prosthetic Engineering, VAPSHCS, 1660 South Columbian Way, Seattle, WA 98195, USA
[c] University of Washington, 1959 Northeast Pacific, Seattle, WA 98195, USA
[d] Department of Orthopaedics and Sports Medicine, Harborview Medical Center, 325 Ninth Avenue, Box 359799, Seattle, WA 98104, USA
* Corresponding author. #1001-328 11th Avenue East, Vancouver, BC V5T4W1, Canada.
E-mail address: kapostle@me.com

Foot Ankle Clin N Am 17 (2012) 1–11
doi:10.1016/j.fcl.2011.11.001
1083-7515/12/$ – see front matter © 2012 Elsevier Inc. All rights reserved.

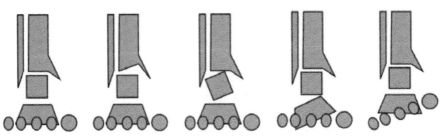

Fig. 1. Varus deformities of the foot and ankle. Left to right; normal, varus of the tibial plafond, varus tilt of the talus in the mortise, varus hindfoot, and forefoot varus.

biomechanical limitations to the foot and ankle. This article provides an overview of the anatomic variations seen with varus deformity of the ankle and foot.

FOREFOOT-DRIVEN HINDFOOT VARUS

Forefoot-driven hindfoot varus refers to a flexible hindfoot that is capable of neutral position but is driven into varus to compensate for a plantarflexed first ray. This condition is clinically demonstrable by Coleman block testing, in which the hindfoot position is observed to correct with posting of the lateral column of the foot.[1] Common soft tissue pathologies resulting in forefoot-driven hindfoot varus are listed in **Box 1**. In addition to causing a varus hindfoot position, these conditions are also associated with a cavus, or high-arched, foot. The cavovarus deformity clinically observed is caused by overdrive of the extrinsic musculature of the foot in an agonist-antagonist pattern. These deformities typically begin as correctable; however, with time, the soft tissues become contracted and fibrotic and the deformity may become fixed. The typical pattern of muscle imbalance is due to overdrive of the peroneus longus and tibialis posterior relative to the antagonizing tibialis anterior and peroneus brevis (**Fig. 2**). Charcot-Marie-Tooth is one of the more frequent causes of forefoot-driven hindfoot varus. In this condition, a common finding is relative weakness of the peroneus brevis and tibialis anterior, with sparing of the peroneus longus and tibialis posterior.[2]

Box 1
Muscle imbalance and soft tissue pathologies resulting in forefoot-driven hindfoot varus

Charcot-Marie-Tooth and other hereditary sensory motor neuropathies

Idiopathic overdrive of tibialis posterior or peroneus longus

Spinal tumors

Paralytic muscle imbalance

Spinal dysraphism

Post compartment syndrome

Cerebral palsy

Stroke

Plantar fascia contracture (plantar fibromatosis)

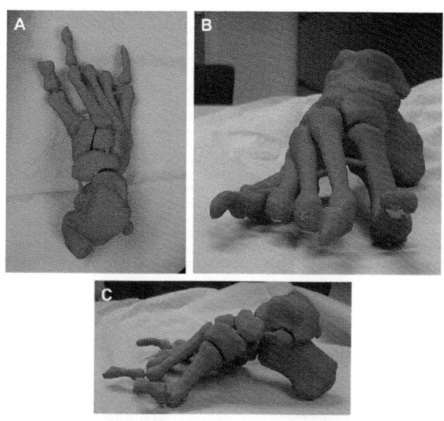

Fig. 2. The cavovarus foot modeled from computed tomographic scan of a patient with a severe deformity. Viewed from above (*A*), note the adduction of the midfoot and forefoot and the supinated midfoot and hindfoot. Viewed from front to back (*B*), the hindfoot varus and reciprocal forefoot valgus may be seen. Viewed from the medial side (*C*), plantarflexion of the first ray is evident, as well as a shortened distance between the calcaneal tuberosity and the first metatarsal head and superior displacement of the navicular as well as dorsal subluxation of the MTP joints.

The tibialis posterior has a broad insertion plantarmedially at the navicular tuberosity and then fans out plantarly over the cuneiforms, cuboid, and base of the second, third, and fourth metatarsals. The tibialis posterior acts to cause inversion and adduction of the midfoot relative to the tibia. The peroneus longus inserts on the base of the first metatarsal and cuneiform as well as the lateral metatarsal neck and acts to plantarflex the first ray. The clinical consequence of an overactive tibialis posterior and peroneus longus is forefoot eversion and midfoot inversion and adduction (see **Fig. 2**).

The over-pull of the tibialis posterior and peroneus longus elevate the medial longitudinal arch and shorten the medial column. This deformity increases the distance between the navicular and the floor and decreases the distance between the calcaneal tuberosity and the first metatarsal head. This change leads to a contracted plantar fascia, which further exacerbates plantarflexion of the first ray via the windlass mechanism.

The weak tibialis anterior cannot dorsiflex the ankle against the strong gastrocsoleus complex, and the extensor hallucis longus and extensor digitorum communis will be recruited as secondary dorsiflexors of the ankle, causing hyperextension of the hallux and lesser toe metatarsophalangeal (MTP) joints. Weakness of the intrinsic muscles of the foot leads to dynamic overdrive of the long toe flexors and extensors, exacerbating the MTP hyperextension and causing interphalangeal flexion. If left uncorrected, this deformity may lead to dorsal dislocation of the MTPs. This dislocation, along with the contracted plantar fascia and shortened medial column, pulls the plantar fat pad proximally and transfers the weight-bearing axis to the metatarsal heads (see **Fig. 2**).

In more severe neuromuscular conditions, the muscle imbalance is easily recognized and the associated clinical deformity can be quite severe.[3] In the more subtle idiopathic cavus foot it is important to look for dynamic long peroneal overdrive.[4] This deformity may not be evident in static stance; however, it may be noted clinically by relative increased plantarflexion of the first ray with resisted plantarflexion of the forefoot when seated. This response can be elicited by asking the patient to forcibly plantarflex the forefoot against the resistance of the examiner's thumbs placed under the first and fifth metatarsal heads. The examiner will note a more forcible plantarflexion of the first

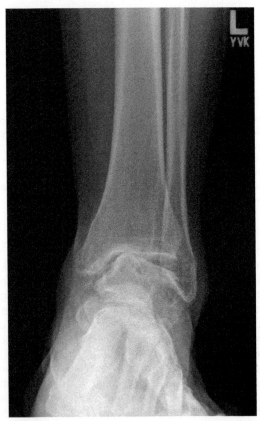

Fig. 3. Varus ankle arthritis following prolonged uncorrected cavovarus secondary to a neuromuscular condition.

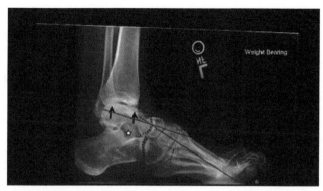

Fig. 4. A cavovarus foot in a patient with a neuromuscular disorder. Note the widened sinus tarsi (*star*), double density of the talar dome (*arrows*), break in the cyma line (*hashed lines*), posterior position of the fibula, superior position of the navicular relative to the cuboid, and a break in the talo–first metatarsal angle (*red lines*).

relative to the fifth metatarsal head resulting in forefoot valgus with plantarflexion. Alternatively, the examiner may ask the patient to evert the hindfoot against resistance. The examiner will note plantarflexion of the first ray as the peroneus longus overpowers the peroneus brevis.

Persistent hindfoot varus deformity may ultimately lead to contracture of the medial soft tissues including the talonavicular capsule, spring ligament, and deltoid complex. As the soft tissue contractures become fixed, rebalancing the muscle function across the ankle and foot becomes insufficient in terms of correcting the foot position.

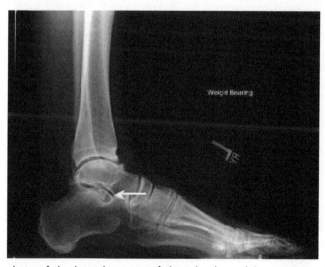

Fig. 5. Osteophyte of the lateral process of the talus (*arrow*) in a patient with a subtle hindfoot varus.

ANATOMIC ABNORMALITIES IN THE NEUROMUSCULAR CAVOVARUS FOOT

In the extremity with a cavovarus position secondary to muscle imbalance, many alterations in the osseous anatomy may be observed. These alterations are discussed from proximal to distal.

At the ankle joint, the talus may be seen to tilt into varus in the mortise. This tilt is a late finding with contracture of the medial soft tissue structures of the foot and ankle. The goal is to correct the muscle imbalance and foot misalignment prior to varus alignment at the ankle, which will cause altered joint reaction forces and ultimate degenerative changes at the medial plafond (**Fig. 3**).

The over-pull of the tibialis posterior and peroneus longus results in inversion at the subtalar joint. This result can be seen on lateral foot radiograph as a widened sinus tarsi, a double density of the talar body, and a break in the cyma line as the calcaneus translates inferior and medial beneath the talus (**Fig. 4**). With time an osteophyte may develop along the lateral process of the talus, which becomes a mechanical block to eversion of the hindfoot and must be removed to determine if the hindfoot position will correct once the pull of the deforming forces has been removed intraoperatively (**Fig. 5**). On the anteroposterior (AP) radiograph, supination of the hindfoot is seen as a narrowing of the talocalcaneal angle and a break in the cyma line (**Fig. 6**).

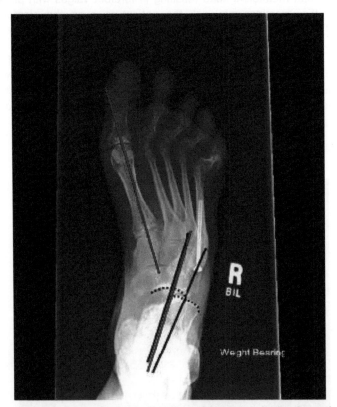

Fig. 6. A neuromuscular cavus foot, AP view. Note the narrowed talocalcaneal angle (*solid lines*), break in the cyma line (*hashed lines*), break in the talo–first metatarsal angle (*red lines*) stacking of the metatarsals, adduction of the midfoot, fifth metatarsal hypertrophy, and screw fixating an old stress fracture of the fifth metatarsal.

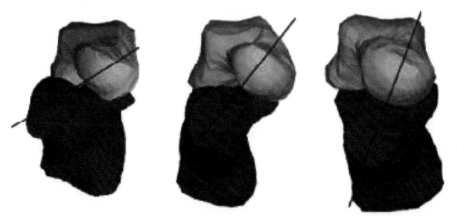

Fig. 7. Position of Chopart joint in hindfoot valgus (*left*), neutral (*middle*) and varus (*right*). The red line approximates the combined axes of the talonavicular and calcaneocuboid joints. Note the more vertical (inverted) position of joint axis in the varus hindfoot. As Chopart joint becomes more vertical, translational motion is blocked and the foot is less able to absorb and dissipate body weight forces.

The inverted subtalar joint causes a reciprocal supination of the Chopart joint, causing the cuboid to be plantarly translated relative to the navicular instead of lateral to it. This position of the Chopart joint makes the foot a more rigid structure that is unable to evert during stance and less able to absorb and dissipate body weight during gait[5] (**Fig. 7**).

The dorsal position of the navicular relative to the cuboid dictates the cascade of the metatarsals, causing a stacking of the metatarsals and overloading of the lateral border of the foot. This deformity can be seen radiographically as a relative hypertrophy or even stress fractures of the lateral rays (see **Fig. 6**). The over-pull of the tibialis posterior adducts and inverts the midfoot and the peroneus longus plantar-flexes the first metatarsal leading to a break in the talo–first metatarsal angle on both AP and lateral radiographs (see **Figs. 4** and **6**).

INTRINSIC VARUS

Intrinsic hindfoot varus refers to a hindfoot position that is fixed in varus because of the anatomy of the bones or joints (**Box 2**). Intrinsic varus may or may not be associated with a cavus foot, because the forefoot will attempt to establish a plantigrade position with respect to the hindfoot. Primary bony pathology resulting in a varus ankle and hindfoot is discussed from proximal to distal.

Most proximally, the orientation of the plafond has a direct relationship to the position of the ankle and hindfoot. The ankle and subtalar joint positions are intimately related because deformity in one causes a compensatory deformity in the other as the foot attempts to establish a plantigrade position underneath the mechanical weight-bearing axis of the extremity. A mobile or hypermobile subtalar joint can compensate for a more proximal deformity, whereas a subtalar joint with more limited motion cannot compensate and will assume the deformity created more proximally. In other words, in a varus plafond, the hindfoot position can be within normal limits if the subtalar joint has sufficient eversion. If not, the hindfoot will also be in varus. Conversely, a valgus plafond may be associated with a compensatory hindfoot varus

---

Box 2
Primary osseous causes of intrinsic hindfoot-driven hindfoot varus

Distal tibial varus or valgus

Varus tilt of talus in mortise (lateral ligament instability)

Varus talar malunion

Varus calcaneal malunion

Varus subtalar joint axis

Excessive tibial external rotation

Tarsal coalition

---

position if the subtalar joint is mobile and assumes a maximally inverted position **(Fig. 8)**. It is important to recognize these deformities and correct the plafond alignment prior to attempting to correct the varus hindfoot position and midfoot and forefoot misalignment.

It is also important to consider the rotational profile of the extremity because excessive tibial external rotation may contribute to a cavovarus deformity.[6] This deformity has been observed to be an adaptive foot position in an active attempt by the individual to improve the line of progression of the foot from its externally rotated position by supinating the subtalar joint and activating the tibialis posterior to adduct the midfoot. Other primary anatomic abnormalities leading to a hindfoot-driven

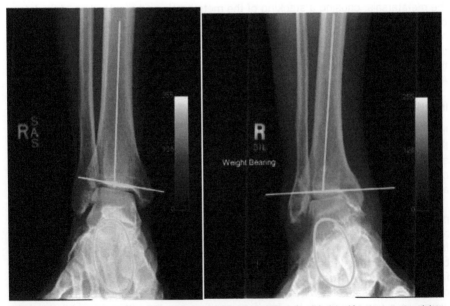

Fig. 8. Distal tibial valgus (*left*) and varus (*right*) associated with hindfoot varus position. Straight green lines approximate the distal tibial plafond alignment. The green ovals denote the longitudinal axis of the calcaneal tuberosity.

hindfoot varus foot position may include varus malunion of a talar neck fracture or calcaneal fracture and tarsal coalition.

In a patient with hindfoot varus and no clinical evidence of muscle imbalance and a normal plafond alignment, the authors have found it important to look at the coronal plane axis of the subtalar joint. The authors routinely obtain weight-bearing computed tomographic scans in patients presenting with varus deformities of the foot and ankle and have found the coronal alignment of the subtalar joint relative to the dome of the talus to be excessively varus in some patients (**Fig. 9**A). This misalignment is

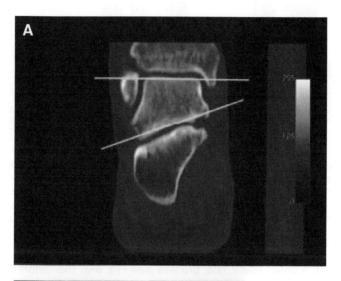

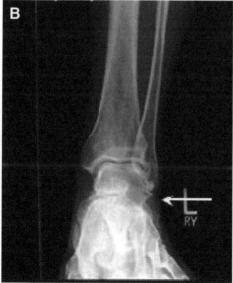

Fig. 9. Varus subtalar joint axis as seen on weight-bearing computed tomographic image (*A*). Note the broad lateral process of the talus and that the subtalar joint cannot be seen laterally on the AP view (*B, arrow*).

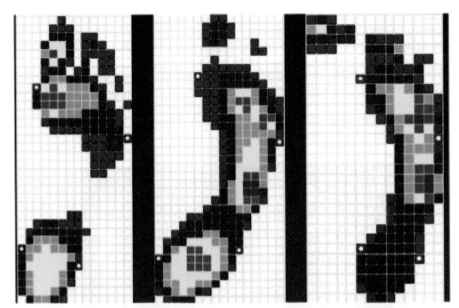

Fig. 10. Pressure data from three different cavovarus feet. Far left: subtle forefoot-driven hindfoot varus showing increased pressures under the first metatarsal head. The middle image shows more severe hindfoot rotation and calcaneal pitch resulting in increased heel pressures and overloading of the lateral border of the foot. Far right shows and extreme equinocavovarus foot in which all the weight is centered on the lateral border of the foot.

associated with a broad lateral talar process (see **Fig. 9**A). This deformity can also been seen on the AP view of the ankle because the subtalar joint cannot be fully appreciated laterally (see **Fig. 9**B). Clinically, patients are found to have a normal overall range of motion of the subtalar joint; however, they will demonstrate excessive inversion and eversion typically not past neutral.

BIOMECHANICAL IMPLICATIONS

The importance of recognizing the cavus abnormality is that it renders the foot more rigid that the normal foot.[5] In the midstance phase of gait, the normal hindfoot will assume an everted position unlocking the subtalar joint allowing for stress absorption throughout the foot. When the hindfoot varus is fixed, the Chopart joint cannot function, and the stress absorption capability of the foot is lost. This result has been shown to lead to overload phenomenon in the foot, specifically under the first metatarsal head and the lateral border of the foot.[7,8] This deformity has specific importance in diabetic patients in whom areas of overload are susceptible to ulceration and the potentially devastating complications that are associated with diabetic ulcerations (**Fig. 10**).[9] Also prolonged varus of the hindfoot causes contracture of the medial soft tissues, causing increased anteromedial ankle joint pressure and subsequent varus ankle arthritis, for which the surgical solutions are less reliable.

SUMMARY

In summary, varus deformity of the foot and ankle encompasses a spectrum of deformities from mild to severe. The cause of this deformity may be bone, muscle imbalance, or a combination of both. Surgical intervention should be planned only after the patient's anatomy is understood. Uncorrected symptomatic varus deformities may have significant consequences on gait kinematics and foot biomechanics.

REFERENCES

1. Coleman SS, Chesnut WJ. A simple test for hindfoot flexibility in the cavovarus foot. Clin Orthop 1977;123:60-2.
2. Sabir M, Lyttle D. Pathogenesis of pes cavus in Charcot-Marie tooth disease. Clin Orthop 1983;175:173-8.
3. Younger AS, Hansen ST. Adult cavovarus foot. J Am Acad Orthop Surg 2005;13(5): 302-15.
4. Chilvers M, Manoli A. The subtle cavus foot and association with ankle instability and lateral foot overload. Foot Ankle Clin 2008;13(2):315-24.
5. Aminian A, Sangeorzan BJ. The anatomy of cavus foot deformity. Foot Ankle Clin 2008;13(2):191-8.
6. Hansen ST, The cavovarus/supinated foot deformity and external tibial torsion: the role of the posterior tibial tendon. Foot Ankle Clin 2008;13(2):325-8.
7. Burns J, Crosbie J, Hunt A, et al. The effect of pes cavus on foot pain and plantar pressure. Clin Biomech 2005;20:877-82.
8. Ledoux WR, Shofer JB, Ahroni JH, et al. Biomechanical differences among pes cavus, neutrally aligned, and pes planus feet in subjects with diabetes. Foot Ankle Int 2003;24(11):845-50.
9. Ledoux WR, Shofer JB, Smith DG, et al. Relationship between foot type, foot deformity, and ulcer occurrence in the high-risk diabetic foot. J Rehabil Res Dev 2005;42(5):665-72.

Examination of the Varus Ankle, Foot, and Tibia

Gowreeson Thevendran, FRCS (Tr & Ortho)[a],
Alastair S. Younger, MD, ChB, FRCSC[b],*

KEYWORDS

- Varus ankle • Varus foot • Varus tibia
- Foot and ankle examination

Varus malalignment of the distal lower extremity can be a challenging condition to treat. The spectrum of involvement of the cavus foot may range from a mildly elevated longitudinal arch in an otherwise functional foot to completely rigid deformities in patients with secondary arthritis, stress fractures, muscle weakness, and ligamentous insufficiency. Patients often present with pain secondary to increased stresses on one part of the foot.[1] For instance, patients with Charcot-Marie-Tooth disease may overload the lateral border of the foot, the first metatarsal head,[2] or the lateral metatarsal heads. This increased load may result in stress fractures, particularly affecting the fifth metatarsal. In athletes, this foot shape results in increased load on the metatarsal heads and on the calcaneus.[3]

The varus hindfoot may also result in lateral ankle instability with continuous attenuation of the lateral collateral ligaments as a result of the medially displaced moment arm of the Achilles tendon. Distal migration of the metatarsal fad pad from beneath the metatarsal heads results in plantar callosities in association with claw toe deformities. Prolonged weight-bearing on the cavus foot also results in medial ankle overload and the joints of the triple-joint complex (subtalar, talonavicular, and calcaneocuboid joints). The abnormal loading over the medial column results in secondary degenerative change and subsequent varus tilt of the talus and lateral ligament laxity.

The varus tibia may be secondary to a variety of causes including previous fracture, tibial physeal injury, or previous surgery. In an otherwise normal foot, the varus tibia will create a hindfoot varus deformity and pronation of the subtalar joint in most feet. This pronation rotational force is driven from the forefoot to the hindfoot because of

No external source of funding for this article.
The authors have nothing to disclose.
[a] Foot and Ankle Surgery, St. Paul's Hospital, 1081 Burrard Street, Vancouver, BC V6Z 1Y6, Canada
[b] Department of Orthopaedics, University of British Columbia, British Columbia's Foot and Ankle Clinic, St. Pauls Hospital, 560 1144 Burrard Street, Vancouver, BC V6Z 2A5, Canada
* Corresponding author.
E-mail address: asyounger@telus.net

Foot Ankle Clin N Am 17 (2012) 13–20
doi:10.1016/j.fcl.2011.11.006
1083-7515/12/$ – see front matter © 2012 Elsevier Inc. All rights reserved.

the mechanical necessity for the forefoot to become plantigrade on the ground. Clinically, this mechanism may manifest as lateral column overload, subtalar joint instability, or sinus tarsi impingement.[4]

CLINICAL ANATOMY

The term *cavus* describes the shape of the foot that includes a higher than average arch.[5] This arch may be secondary to a high pitch angle of the hindfoot, excessive plantarflexion of the forefoot, or excessive bend in the midfoot. In extreme cases this shape may be driven by a narrow talocalcaneal angle and result in complex torsional changes of the midfoot. The components of cavus are increased pitch and varus of the hindfoot, plantarflexion of the midfoot, and varus and adduction of the forefoot.[6] This high arch and varus alignment can be from rigid hindfoot anatomy in the form of abnormal shape and relationship of the talus and calcaneus. Conversely, high arch and varus alignment may also be from a flexible hindfoot that is a secondary deformity resulting from a plantarflexed midfoot and forefoot.

There is a distinction within a cavus deformity that is determined by whether the cavus is driven by forefoot deformity (flexible cavus) or by a hindfoot deformity (fixed cavus). Forefoot-driven cavus is secondary to a relatively plantarflexed first metatarsal head relative to the lesser metatarsals. Thus, when the forefoot contacts the ground, the plantarflexed first ray drives the midfoot dorsally and into varus. This deformity drives the hindfoot into varus as long as the triple joint is flexible. Conversely, hindfoot varus and a high arch may be by themselves attributable to the structure of the hindfoot. Abnormal bony anatomy of the talus or calcaneus may result in an increased pitch angle. Previous trauma may affect talar neck alignment, resulting in varus or adduction.[7]

CLINICAL EXAMINATION

When evaluating a patient with a cavovarus foot deformity, it is important to establish the underlying cause for the condition. The key to proper evaluation is to appreciate the individuality of patients with this condition. The examining physician should above all know the area of maximum tenderness after completing physical examination and diagnose the pathologic condition limiting function. The relationship to the foot mechanics can then be hypothesized, and the correction required guides the treatment plan.

Inspection

Clinical examination should begin with exposing the limb to waist level. The patient should be examined walking and standing, where limb alignment and the weight-bearing posture of the foot and ankle can be assessed. Gait abnormalities may be complex. Swing phase on one side is watched first, then stance phase, and the observation is repeated for the opposite side and continued until the deficits in gait are clear to the examiner. The patient is asked to toe-walk and heel-walk. Failure to toe-walk may indicate weakness, pain, or instability. Failure to heel-walk may indicate contractures or weakness of the extensors.

Gait assessment is pivotal to unmask subtle deformities and further analyze loading patterns. The presence of foot drop, hyperextension of the great or lesser toes, and malalignment of the forefoot or hindfoot may be better appreciated during the swing phase of the gait cycle. Stance phase is analyzed from heel-strike to toe-off. Adaptive gait patterns and the position of calluses should reinforce the observations of gait.

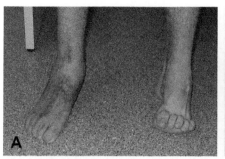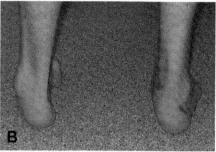

Fig. 1. A patient after a cavus reconstruction on the right and preoperative on the left. The anterior view (*A*) with the internal rotation of the forefoot on the left, claw toes, plantar-flexed first ray, and hindfoot varus with a peek-a-boo heel sign. The posterior view (*B*) shows the hindfoot varus and the internal rotation of the forefoot. This deformity is corrected on the operative side.

While standing, the hindfoot and forefoot position are observed. Muscle wasting and overall limb alignment are observed. The shape of the foot, including the presence or absence of clawing of the toes and the presence or absence of a varus hindfoot, must be noted (**Fig. 1**). The peek-a-boo heel sign may be observed when viewing the patient from the front with the feet aligned straight (**Fig. 2**). First described in 1993 in an article describing lower extremity contractures, this test can be sensitive even for identifying the subtle cavus foot.[8] When viewed from the front, the varus heel will be visualized medially in a cavus foot.[9] Conversely, physiologic heel valgus will not display this characteristic. The amount of heel visualized medially should be compared with the contralateral side. A false-positive peek-a-boo sign may be caused by a very large heel pad or significant metatarsus adductus.[10]

Once sitting, callus formation may be observed in the areas of load (**Fig. 3**). The hindfoot position is documented by comparing the relationship between the

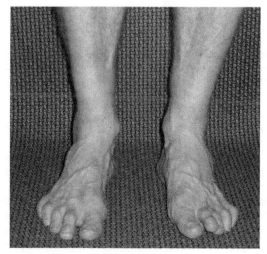

Fig. 2. The peek-a-boo heel sign in a subtle cavus foot.

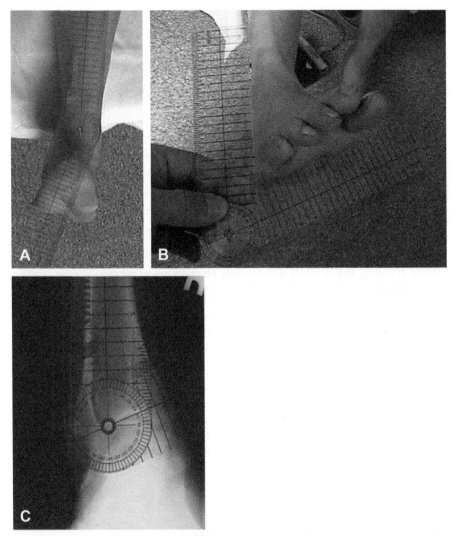

Fig. 3. A patient with hindfoot varus measured at 20° with a goniometer (*A*). The forefoot has a similar position of varus on the long axis of the limb, showing that the forefoot is neutral on the hindfoot (*B*). The deformity in this patient exists at the ankle joint (*C*).

tuberosity of the calcaneus against a line visualized from the center of the knee through the center of the ankle. This position can be reproduced on the operating table to determine hindfoot correction. A tuberosity medial to the long axis of the leg reflects hindfoot varus, and lateral to the midline is in valgus (rarely seen in the cavus foot) (**Fig. 3**).

The relationship of the forefoot to the hindfoot should be documented. The hindfoot and midfoot are placed in the neutral position and the relationship of the forefoot is observed. The forefoot to hindfoot position can be described in one of three ways. A plantigrade (neutral) forefoot occurs when both the planes of the forefoot and hindfoot are parallel to each other. If the lateral aspect of the foot is

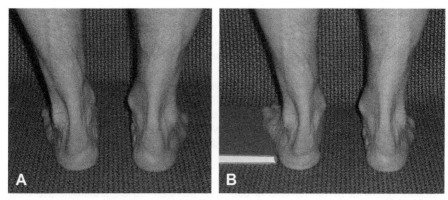

Fig. 4. The Coleman block test. The hindfoot varus that is present (*A*) is corrected after the block is placed under the lateral border of the foot (*B*), indicating that the hindfoot is flexible and the forefoot is plantarflexed.

more plantarflexed than the medial aspect, this is termed *forefoot varu*s (supinated position). This deformity occurs in clubfoot and after talar neck fracture, or deformity within the ankle. Conversely, if the medial aspect is more plantarflexed, this is termed *forefoot valgus* (pronated position). This deformity occurs more often in neurologic causes.

The relation of the forefoot to the hindfoot may be supple or rigid, an important finding to document when considering surgery to create a plantigrade foot. A fixed forefoot deformity will not permit the foot to become plantigrade once the heel is placed in a neutral position, and a surgical procedure, likely a derotation and fusion at the level of the Chopart joints, may be required in order to realign the forefoot onto the hindfoot.

The forefoot position needs to be assessed in the transverse plane. This position can be indexed from the axis of the femur with the knee flexed to 90°. If the forefoot is medial to this line, then the foot is internally rotated (adducted). If external to this plane, the foot is externally rotated or abducted. This deformity is rarely seen in the cavus foot. The internal rotation of the forefoot medializes the joint reaction force in the ankle significantly. Palpation of the transmalleolar axis will determine if this deformity is present above the ankle or below the ankle and within the hindfoot.

The sum of the joint reaction force at the ankle will be most medialized with an internally rotated forefoot having the greatest effect, followed by a plantarflexed first ray causing forefoot valgus, and hindfoot varus.

Coleman and Chestnut[11] are acknowledged for presenting perhaps the single most important contribution to the development of a methodical assessment of the cavovarus foot in 1977. In their classic manuscript, they described an elegant but simple method to assess the degree of flexibility of the hindfoot in a patient who has a cavus deformity. The Coleman block test necessitates that a patient stand on a block of wood with the heel and the lateral forefoot supported by the block, which enables the plantarflexed first ray to depress (**Fig. 4**). The examiner, positioned behind the patient, is then able to assess if the hindfoot deformity is corrected. If the maneuver of dropping the first ray over the edge of the block allows for the hindfoot to correct to a valgus position, the hindfoot is flexible. Conversely, if the correction of the varus hindfoot is not observed, the hindfoot is rigid. This deformity is often referred to as forefoot-driven hindfoot varus. From a treatment perspective, this single discriminant finding may help distinguish those patients with a supple hindfoot who would benefit from an orthosis against those with a fixed hindfoot deformity who may require surgery. Surgically, this procedure is likely to entail correction of the varus deformity (eg, calcaneal osteotomy or subtalar fusion) and a dorsiflexion osteotomy of the first ray.

Peroneus longus overdrive may also be identified. The examiner places one thumb under the first metatarsal head and the other thumb beneath the remaining metatarsal heads. The patient is then asked to plantarflex the foot into the examiner's thumbs. With peroneus longus overdrive, more force will be felt under the first metatarsal head as compared with the lateral metatarsal heads.[12]

Palpation

Establishing points of tenderness is useful to correlate to an anatomic site of a pathologic condition. In the varus tibia, medial joint line tenderness across the knee may be an early sign of degenerative joint disease and/or meniscal abnormality. In the varus ankle, medial compartment overload may manifest as medial joint line tenderness or anteromedial ankle joint impingement. Attenuation of the lateral collateral ligament may result in tenderness along the calcaneofibular ligament or the anterior talofibular ligament. Tendons are palpated to ascertain if they are a source of pain. Nodularity and thickening of the tendon sheath may be suggestive of tendinosis.

Forefoot pain may result in metatarsalgia or first metatarsal head overload. Palpation of the position of the metatarsal heads and determination of pain will help the surgeon identify the metatarsals carrying load. Calluses may be present and painful over the interphalangeal joints.

Stress fractures can occur in the metatarsal shafts. Pain will be localized over the area of fracture and can exist in the second, fourth, or fifth metatarsal shafts.

Pain on palpation can exist in the midfoot over arthritic joints. Increased skin temperature can allow an arthritic joint to be localized, as well as precise localization of pain.

Movement

The function of various joints can be observed from the plane of their primary motions. For the ankle joint, this function is plantarflexion and dorsiflexion with a small contribution of internal-extremal rotation and varus-valgus through the entire range of motion in the sagittal plane. Side-to-side comparisons are more valuable than absolute ranges.

For the subtalar joint, the plane of motion is a modified coronal plane that is rotated externally (on average 67°) and plantarflexed (average 48° from the vertical). At the midtarsal joints, the primary plane of motion is abduction and adduction, with a lesser degree of plantarflexion and dorsiflexion occurring. There should be minimal motion at the navicular cuneiform and tarsometatarsal joints. During assessment of range of motion, the passive and active arcs of motion of all major articulations of both feet are checked for limitation of motion, fixed or flexible deformities, painful arc of motion, and crepitus.

Each joint should be isolated in turn, the surrounding bones moved, and then the joint lines palpated to assess the source of discomfort.

Special Tests

The Achilles tendon is tested for tightness with the knee both flexed and extended. A lack of change in equinus between the two positions may indicate a mechanical block to ankle dorsiflexion from a tight posterior capsule or anterior impinging osteophytes. Rarely, an isolated contracture of the soleus may cause restriction of ankle dorsiflexion with the knee in both flexion and extension. Equinus with the knee straight but increased dorsiflexion with the knee flexed indicates a tight gastrocnemius muscle.

The degree of lateral talar tilt should be assessed with the ankle in full plantarflexion and neutral dorsiflexion. The foot is inverted forcibly, and any excessive talar tilt may be suggestive of lateral ligamentous injury. With the foot in plantarflexion the anterior talofibular ligament is tested, and with the ankle in neutral dorsiflexion the calcaneofibular ligament is assessed.[13] The anterior drawer test is performed as a rotational motion. The ankle is held in slight plantarflexion and the calcaneus is pulled anteriorly and internally rotated while holding the tibia with the opposite hand, and one finger is held over the anterior lateral corner of the ankle palpating the talus. Forward translation of more than 3 to 4 mm is indicative of laxity. A fixed varus deformity of the foot and ankle may result in ankle instability because the plantarflexed first metatarsal forces the calcaneus to invert. The peroneals may be unable to compensate because of weakness, pain, or rupture.[14] The lateral collateral ligaments may become deficient through the same process.

Neurovascular Exam

Function and strength of all muscle groups should be documented, because these tests allow an assessment of progression of the disease over time and help the surgeon best understand the options for surgical reconstruction. The strength of each muscle is tested against active resistance applied by the examiner, and the results are graded using the Medical Research Council (MRC) scale. The grading in this scale ranges from 0 to 5: grade 0, no contraction; grade 1, flicker or trace of contraction; grade 2, active movement with gravity eliminated; grade 3, active movement against gravity; grade 4, active movement against gravity and resistance; and grade 5, normal power. When performing muscle transfers as part of a surgical reconstruction of the varus distal lower extremity, accurate documentation of individual muscle agonist and antagonists MRC strength grades is pivotal to ensure deforming forces are recognized and the final muscle imbalance is dealt with correctly.

A thorough neurovascular examination is important both as a diagnostic and prognostic measure. Sensory modalities may be affected selectively (posterior column disease) or globally (post compartment syndrome). An astute recognition of the pattern of loss (ie, stocking distribution, peripheral nerve distribution, or radicular pattern) may help consolidate a provisional diagnosis.

Semmes-Weinstein monofilaments may be used to ascertain the degree of sensory loss. The Tinel test should be performed along the course of nerves and painful scars. Finally, pulsations of the dorsalis pedis and posterior tibial vessels must be documented at first consultation.

SUMMARY

A detailed clinical examination is an essential component in the assessment of the cavus foot. A complex interaction of pathologic conditions can only be assessed completely with physical examination. Imaging such as computed tomography or magnetic resonance imaging (MRI) may confound the physician, such as in anterior talofibular ligament tears on MRI while the ankle is stable or arthritic joints that are asymptomatic but abnormal on imaging.

At the end of the day, the physical examination supersedes all other investigations. After investigations have been performed, the patient needs to be reviewed and the results interpreted in light of the clinical findings. At this point the examiner will be able to determine what is significant and decide on an appropriate treatment plan.

REFERENCES

1. Younger AS, Hansen ST. Adult cavovarus foot. J Am Acad Orthop Surg 2005;13: 302–15.
2. Alexander IJ, Johnson KA. Assessment and management of pes cavus in Charcot-Marie-Tooth disease. Clin Orthop 1989;246:273–81.
3. Sneyers CJ, Lysens R, Feys H, et.al. Influence of malalignment of feet on the plantar pressure pattern in running. Foot Ankle Int 1995;16:624–32.
4. Silver RL, de la Garza J, Rang M. The myth of muscle balance. A study of relative strengths and excursions of normal muscles about the foot and ankle. J Bone Joint Surg Br 1985;67:432–7.
5. Aminian A, Sangeorzan B. The Anatomy of cavus foot deformity. Foot Ankle Clin 2008;13:191–8.
6. Holmes JR, Hansen ST. Foot and ankle manifestations of Charcot-Marie-Tooth disease. Foot Ankle 1993:14(8);476–86.
7. Canale ST, Kelly FB Jr. Fractures of the neck of the talus. Long-term evaluation of seventy-one cases. J Bone Joint Surg Am 1978;60:143–56.
8. Manoli A II, Smith DG, Hansen ST Jr. Scarred muscle excision for the treatment of established ischemic contracture of the lower extremity. Clin Orthop 1977;123:60–2.
9. Beals TC, Manoli A II. The peak-a-boo heel sign in the evaluation of hindfoot varus. Foot 1996;6:205–6.
10. Desai S, Grierson R, Manoli A II. The Cavus foot in athletes: fundamentals of examination and treatment. Oper Tech Sports Med 2010;18:27–33.
11. Coleman SS, Chestnut WJ. A simple test for hindfoot flexibility in the cavovarus foot. Clin Orthop Relat Res 1977;123:60–2.
12. Bordelon RL. Practical guide to foot orthoses. J Musculoskel Med 1989;6:71–87.
13. Jahss MN. Evaluation of the cavus foot for orthopaedic treatment. Clin Orthop Relat Res 1983;181:52–63.
14. Medhat MA, Kantz H. Neuropathic ankle joint in Charcot-Marie-Tooth disease after triple arthrodesis of the foot. Orthop Rev 1988;17:873–80.

Varus Ankle and Osteochondral Lesions of the Talus

Mark E. Easley, MD[a],*, J. Carr Vineyard, MD[b]

KEYWORDS
- Malalignment of the ankle • Osteochondral lesion of the talus
- Supramalleolar osteotomy • Varus ankle

To our knowledge, little is reported about the management of the patients with combined symptomatic osteochondral lesions of the talus (OLT) and varus ankle malalignment.[1] Treatment strategies for symptomatic OLTs are relatively well described in the orthopaedic literature.[2–13] While less defined than the surgical management of OLTs, realignment procedures for the varus ankle and hindfoot have also been studied and reported in some detail, albeit with a focus on management of ankle arthritis.[14–26] In this article we review practical concepts from the orthopaedic literature that may be applied when treating patients with concomitant OLTs and varus ankles malalignment.

Our review analyzes 2 relatively well-described but distinct treatment algorithms in the orthopedic foot and ankle literature: (1) Surgical management of varus ankle and hindfoot alignment and (2) operative treatment of OLTs. We attempt to extrapolate relevant information from the literature should these 2 distinct entities occur in combination in a single patient.

We are uncertain if the natural history of ankles malaligned in varus is one that leads to development of a medial OLT and/or medial talar dome and tibial plafond osteoarthritis. Most investigators agree that continued eccentric loading of the medial aspect of the ankle creates greater than physiologic contact stresses on the medial ankle's articular surfaces,[16,27,28] and some authors extrapolate that these increased contact stresses lead to focal ankle osteochondral defects and arthritis.[27] In select cases, varus ankle alignment may be associated with chronic lateral ankle ligament instability, which may contribute to eccentric joint loading.[29–33]

What is the pain generator in an OLT?[34] Theoretically, mechanical overload from eccentric contact stresses on the OLT may increase OLT-related symptoms. To our knowledge, the majority of symptomatic OLTs exist with physiologic ankle alignment and thus simply treating the malalignment in isolation without directly treating of the OLT will most likely not relieve symptoms adequately. In our opinion, simultaneous or staged treatment of the OLT and ankle malalignment is warranted. By creating a more physiologic tibiotalar load distribution, realignment osteotomies with or without lateral

[a] Department of Orthopaedic Surgery, Duke University Medical Center, 4709 Creekstone Drive, Box 2950, Durham, NC 27703, USA
[b] W.B. Carrell Memorial Clinic, 9301 North Central Expressway, Suite 400, Dallas, TX 75231, USA
* Corresponding author.

Foot Ankle Clin N Am 17 (2012) 21–38
doi:10.1016/j.fcl.2011.11.011
1083-7515/12/$ – see front matter © 2012 Published by Elsevier Inc.
foot.theclinics.com

ankle ligament reconstruction may have a protective effect on the medial ankle carti-lage.[16,29,31,17–19,21,23–26] Realignment osteotomies for varus malalignment tends to relieve symptoms related to associated ankle arthritis even when the ankle arthritis is not treated with a definitive procedure such as arthrodesis or total ankle replace-ment.[14,17,18,26,35] We are uncertain if realignment of varus into a more physiologic position in patients with a concomitant medial OLT obviates the need to directly address the OLT; in our anecdotal experience, we have surgically treated symptomatic OLTs failing nonoperative management and have performed realignment to unload the oper-ated OLT.

COMPARISON WITH SIMILAR CONDITIONS IN THE KNEE

Although the ankle does not have distinct compartments, the medial talar dome—and particularly the medial talar shoulder—may be likened to the medial compartment of the knee. Loosely, treatment principles for medial compartment osteochondral defects or medial unicompartmental arthritis may be extrapolated to the ankle.[36–38] However, we believe that a direct comparison between medial ankle and knee osteochondral defects should not be drawn for the following reasons: (1) Lack of a cruciate ligament system in the ankle, (2) inherent bony and cartilaginous stability of ankle mortise not present in the knee, (3) complexity of the ankle–hindfoot couple in contrast to the single articulation at the knee,[39] and (4) differences in ankle and knee articular cartilage.[33,40,41] Thus, extrapolating treatment experiences for knee varus associated with a medial compartment osteochondral defect to explain treatment of the varus ankle with a medial OLT may not be appropriate.

EVALUATION OF OLT

Once we suspect an OLT based on history and physical examination, we obtain routine weight-bearing ankle radiographs to identify an OLT. Magnetic resonance imaging (MRI) is generally effective in confirming the presence of an OLT and potential associated findings, such as marrow edema, other cartilage defects, lateral ligament attenuation, and tendon abnormalities. We relatively routinely perform a diagnostic (and possibly thera-peutic) ankle corticosteroid injection to confirm intra-articular symptoms. If surgery is considered for the OLT, we recommend computed tomography (CT) to classify and define the dimensions of the OLT.[42] In our experience, MRI displays associated marrow edema and diffuse signal change affiliated with the OLT that may not allow the distinct characterization of the OLT as well as CT. Although arthroscopy may represent the gold standard in evaluation of OLTs,[43] we do not routinely perform diagnostic arthroscopy, given the detailed information gleaned from preoperative MRI and CT.

MANAGEMENT OF OLT

We apply the same treatment strategy to all symptomatic OLTs, irrespective of alignment. Although there may be promising technology on the horizon for manage-ment of OLTs,[44] current treatment strategies have evolved considerably over the last 2 decades.[2] Our simplified surgical treatment algorithm for a medial OLT that we employ loosely adheres to that recommended by most experienced foot and ankle specialists in the United States:

1. OLT without subchondral cyst: Arthroscopic debridement and microfracture.[3,4,45]
2. OLT with small subchondral cyst (surface area <10 × 10 mm and depth ≤7 mm): Consider arthroscopic debridement and microfracture for smaller cysts.[46,47]
3. OLT with intact cartilage cap but subchondral cyst: Arthroscopic inspection to ensure cartilage cap/subchondral bone is intact and retrograde curettage and bone grafting of the cyst.[11,48]

4. Large OLT with a large, contained subchondral cyst: Consider initial arthroscopic debridement but a low threshold for open osteochondral transfer.[5,12]
5. OLT with voluminous subchondral defect involving the talar shoulder: Structural allograft reconstruction of the medial talar dome using a size-matched fresh allograft donor talus.[8–10]

Although we recommend that OLTs be treated the same regardless of ankle alignment, 1 consideration is the medial malleolar osteotomy occasionally required for optimal cartilage repair or reconstruction.[2,5,7,8] Medial malleolar osteotomy must be planned carefully if a concomitant supramalleolar osteotomy is warranted.

Alternate technology may eventually lead to rewriting this treatment algorithm. Although autologous chondrocyte implantation techniques have not been universally accepted for management of OLTs,[49] matrices with autologous chondrocytes or juvenile cartilage cells for implantation into prepared OLTs may ultimately gain wider acceptance and regulatory approval.[44] Eventually, matrices with either cultured or tissue engineered cartilage cells may be implanted arthroscopically, obviating the need for the medial malleolar osteotomy.

EVALUATION OF LIMB ALIGNMENT AND ANKLE STABILITY
Clinical and Radiographic Evaluation

Varus alignment may not be isolated to the ankle and the history and physical examination should include the entire affected extremity, from hip to foot. In cases of prior trauma or surgery proximal to the ankle and/or when the weight-bearing physical examination suggests potential proximal limb deformity, we typically obtain weight-bearing, full-length, hip-to-ankle mechanical axis radiographs. Occasionally, deformity proximal to the ankle joint must be treated to effectively realign the ankle.

In our experience, varus alignment necessitates a comprehensive clinical and radiographic evaluation of the foot, because talar position depends on hindfoot position and the ankle and foot function in concert via the ankle–hindfoot ligamentous couple.[39] Weight-bearing examination of the foot may demonstrate heel varus, cavus, and/or first ray plantarflexion (forefoot-driven hindfoot varus). We recommend that the contribution of the first ray to varus hindfoot position and hindfoot flexibility be assessed using the Coleman Block test.[50] Routine anterior-posterior and lateral foot radiographs generally define a cavus foot posture, particularly in the presence of talo–first metatarsal axis incongruence in both planes.

Despite varus ankle alignment, the hindfoot may be in a compensatory valgus position.[19,51] With ankle realignment from varus to a physiologic position, the ankle–hindfoot ligament couple may correct the hindfoot to its anatomic position. However, occasionally compensatory subtalar valgus position will not correct with ankle realignment, resulting in in greater than physiologic heel valgus and potential subfibular impingement.[19,51] We recommend that preoperative hindfoot position be assessed on weight-bearing Saltzman hindfoot axis views.[52]

Varus alignment may be associated with lateral ankle ligament instability/peroneal tendon attenuation and medial ankle ligament/posterior tibial tendon (PTT) contracture, particularly in an incongruent varus ankle deformity.[17] Some investigators emphasize that ankle malalignment should not be evaluated independent of lateral ankle ligament stability.[17,19] In the patient with varus alignment, we routinely perform anterior drawer testing and evaluate peroneal tendons/muscles with palpation and active eversion against resistance. We assess medial contractures by attempting passive correction of the ankle and hindfoot deformity (**Fig. 1**). Moreover, passive correction from varus to a neutral ankle and hindfoot position, peroneus longus

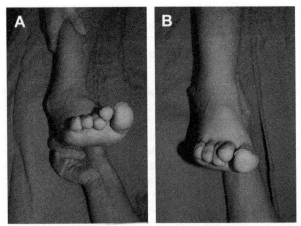

Fig. 1. Clinical examination for passive correction of ankle/hindfoot varus (may be combined with fluoroscopy to more accurately determine if talus can be reduced in the ankle mortise). (*A*) Without valgus/eversion stress. (*B*) With valgus/eversion stress.

contracture may be evidenced with increased first ray plantarflexion or rigidity;[50] in our opinion, a peroneus longus-to-brevis tendon transfer should be considered in this situation. As suggested by several authors, varus alignment may be 1 component of multiplanar deformity,[17,23,25] often associated with concomitant sagittal plane malposition on the lateral radiograph. Congruent varus malalignment may be affiliated with recurvatum deformity; incongruent varus deformity may exist with anterior talar subluxation relative to the tibial plafond.[17,15,23–25]

MRI is rarely indicated in the workup of varus alignment; however, because it may be obtained to further evaluate the OLT, clinical suspicion of peroneal tendon pathology may be confirmed. CT is useful in defining the extent of ankle arthritis and identifying potential hindfoot arthritis; this may have some bearing on surgical management.[2,42] Diffuse ankle arthritis may necessitate alternative procedures to focal management of an OLT and treatment of associated hindfoot arthritis may be warranted to provide the patient with satisfactory relief of symptoms.

MANAGEMENT OF LIMB ALIGNMENT AND ANKLE STABILITY

In our opinion, realignment procedures for correction of varus malalignment associated with OLTs should follow the same treatment recommendations recommended for arthritis in the varus ankle. Although the existing literature lacks a consensus for ankle realignment, several reasonable procedures have been described to treat the symptomatic varus ankle.

Supramalleolar Osteotomy With or Without Fibular Osteotomy

Commonly described supramalleolar osteotomyCommonly described supramalleolar osteotomy techniques to realign the varus ankle are the medial opening and lateral closing wedge osteotomies. One criticism of the lateral closing wedge procedure is that it may lead to limb shortening.[14,26,53] A simultaneous fibular osteotomy is required in all lateral closing wedge osteotomies;[14,26,53] in contrast, for the medial opening wedge procedure, the fibular osteotomy is optional.[16,17,23,54] Alternatively, a coronal plane dome osteotomy may be considered. As for the lateral closing wedge procedure, in our experience the dome osteotomy necessitates performing a simultaneous fibular osteotomy.

To our knowledge, no consensus has been established for when a fibular osteotomy should be performed in conjunction with the medial opening wedge tibial osteotomy. Whereas Lee and Cho[54] reported that the varus ankle may be corrected

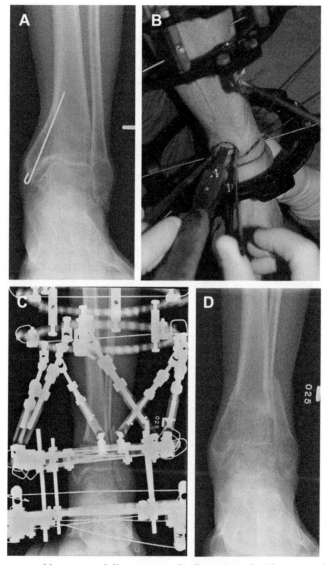

Fig. 2. Congruent ankle varus malalignment gradually corrected with supramalleolar (tibial and fibular) osteotomy (corticotomy) and multiplanar external fixation. (*A*) Preoperative weight-bearing radiograph. (*B*) Intraoperative view of minimally invasive corticotomy. (*C*) Follow-up weight-bearing radiograph of correction using external fixation. (*D*) One-year follow-up weight-bearing radiograph; note correction of varus while maintaining optimal talar position under tibial shaft axis (ie, no translation of talus relative to tibia).

without fibular osteotomy, Takakura colleagues and Stamatis and associates routinely performed fibular osteotomies in all cases.[23–26,53] More recently, Knupp and colleagues,[17] in an elegant investigation describing their classification scheme, suggested that a fibular osteotomy in conjunction with medial opening wedge osteotomy, in their hands, is not routine. These authors explained that once they have completed the medial opening wedge osteotomy in cases of incongruent varus deformity with talar tilt (asymmetric varus deformity, type II according to their classification scheme), they make an intraoperative decision to perform additional procedures, including fibular osteotomy, depending on the residual deformity.[17]

Most commonly, we perform supramalleolar osteotomies with acute deformity correction and internal fixation. However, gradual correction with multiplanar external fixation has also been described.[15] Several authors have suggested that varus ankle alignment is frequently associated with a recurvatum deformity in the sagittal plane, resulting in a relative greater than physiologic anterior slope of the tibial plafond.[16,28,17,23–26] Thus, acute biplanar correction requires a simultaneous medial and anterior opening wedge procedure. Multiplanar external fixation with gradual postoperative biplanar correction after corticotomy may confer an advantage over acute correction with internal fixation in select cases[15] (**Fig. 2**).

Either the combined medial opening wedge supramalleolar and fibular osteotomy or lateral closing wedge supramalleolar osteotomy, if hinged at the apex of the osteotomy, may promote translation of the tibial plafond and talus relative to the tibial shaft axis.[15,26,53] Preoperative planning with reference to the center of rotation and angulation typically allows determination of required compensatory translation to allow the tibial plafond and talus to remain directly under the tibial shaft axis.[15,26,53] Modern multiplanar external fixation, functioning as a virtual hinge, adjusts for potential translation deformity while correcting the angular deformity (see **Fig. 2**).

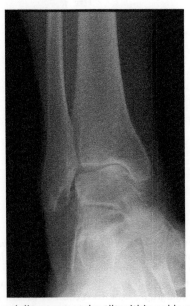

Fig. 3. Incongruent varus malalignment—talar tilt within ankle mortise.

Congruent Versus Incongruent Varus Ankle Alignment

Ankle varus alignment may present in 2 general categories: Congruent (see **Fig. 2**A) or incongruent (**Fig. 3**) deformity, both of which may be associated with an OLT or ankle arthritis and are easily distinguished on standard coronal plane radiographs. A congruent deformity has an anatomically aligned talus and mortise symmetrically tilted into varus secondary to an extra-articular, typically supramalleolar, varus alignment. An incongruent deformity has an asymmetric varus talar tilt within the ankle mortise. Borrowing from what is published about ankle arthritis, these 2 categories are included in classifications of ankle arthritis.[17,23–25] In general, successful outcome is more predictable with realignment for congruent deformity than with incongruent deformity[17,19]; not surprisingly, this experience is what is reported in the total ankle replacement literature.

Varus talar tilt may be managed with supramalleolar osteotomy, but probably most effectively with lesser degrees of talar tilt. Lee and associates[19] suggested that talar tilt of less than 7.3° had a more favorable outcome. Lee and colleague's findings are supported by Tanaka and associates'[25] report that all 12 cases of preoperative talar tilt less than 5° maintained radiographic correction postoperatively, whereas all 7 cases with preoperative talar tilt exceeding 10° did not.[25] However, residual talar tilt noted radiographically does not portend a poor clinical outcome, at least not at intermediate term follow-up.[17] Knupp and co-workers reported that although only 25

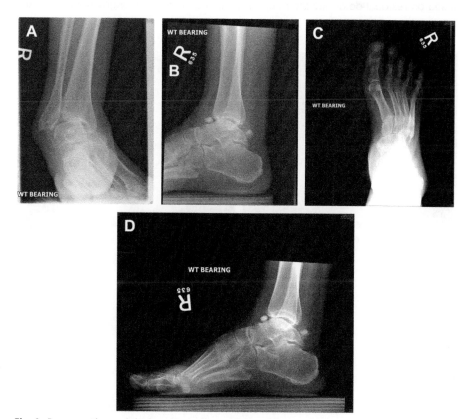

Fig. 4. Preoperative weight-bearing radiographs in a 38 year old male. (*A*) Anterior–posterior (AP) ankle. (*B*) Lateral ankle. (*C*) AP foot. (*D*) Lateral foot.

of 60 ankles with preoperative talar tilt reduced radiographically, the clinical outcome was still improved in the majority of these patients.[17] The authors surmised that realignment may function as an indirect Achilles tendon transfer, redirecting the Achilles tendon's pull on the hindfoot (and thus the talus) into a position that contributes to unloading of the medial ankle joint.

Overcorrection and Compensatory Hindfoot Position and Impingement

Several investigators have recommended overcorrection of varus through the supramalleolar osteotomy into a valgus position.[19,21–25] Whereas some authors report that overcorrection unloads the medial ankle joint more effectively than correction to physiologic alignment, others caution that overcorrection leads to lateral translation of the t bial plaflond and resultant symptomatic lateral impingement.[19] Furthermore, patients with preoperative compensatory hindfoot valgus may be at greater risk for subfibular impingement if they are corrected beyond physiologic ankle realignment.[19,51] Furthermore, supramalleolar osteotomy overcorrection does not lead to improved correction of talar tilt,[17,19] suggesting that additional foot realignment and soft-tissue rebalancing procedures may be warranted in the surgical realignment of varus ankles.[17,19]

ADDITIONAL PROCEDURES TO SUPRAMALLEOLAR OSTEOTOMY

Knupp and associates[17] suggest that the need for additional procedures should be based on residual deformity after supramalleolar osteotomy. Congruent varus ankle

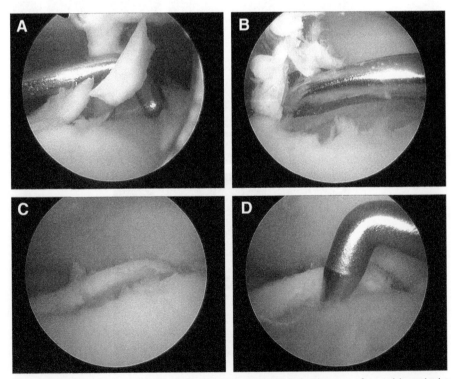

Fig. 5. Arthroscopic views. (*A*) Medial talar dome OLT. (*B*) Debridement of unstable articular cartilage. (*C*) Debrided OLT with stable cartilage rim. (*D*) Microfracture.

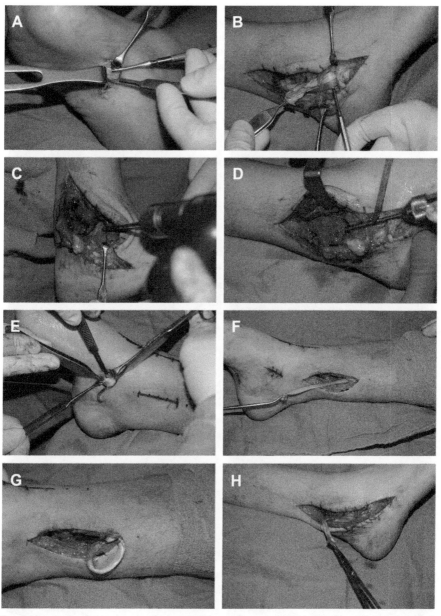

Fig. 6. Surgical management of varus ankle and cavus foot deformity. (*A*) Plantar fascia release. (*B*) Debridement of peroneal tendons and peroneus longus to brevis tendon transfer with residual tendons. (*C, D*) Drill holes for planned allograft lateral ankle ligament reconstruction. (*E–H*) PTT harvest and transfer to lateral foot.

deformity typically can be treated with isolated supramalleolar tibial (and sometimes fibular) osteotomy.[17,19,23–25,54] In contrast, incongruent varus ankle alignment with talar tilt is frequently associated with foot deformity and lateral ankle ligament laxity, prompting consideration of potential calcaneal osteotomy, midfoot osteotomy and/or arthrodesis, and first metatarsal dorsiflexion osteotomy of the first metatarsal.[17,50] Although a preoperative plan for a predicted combination of realignment procedures may be devised, we recommend that residual deformity after supramalleolar osteotomy be assessed intraoperatively under fluoroscopic guidance with talar tilt passively corrected. On occasion, the medial soft tissue contracture is so severe that passive

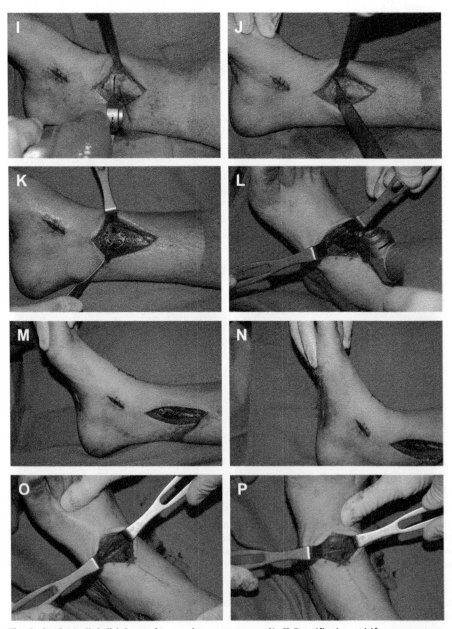

Fig. 6. (*I–K*) Medial tibial opening wedge osteotomy. (*L–P*) Dorsiflexion midfoot osteotomy to correct global cavus deformity.

correction of the residual talar tilt is not possible. In this case, we suggest a judicious medial soft tissue release, including the deltoid ligament, and in severe cases, the PTT. In these severe cavovarus cases, we almost uniformly perform lateral ankle ligament repair/reconstruction and/or peroneus longus-to-brevis transfer after medial soft tissue release. In our experience in patients with severe cavovarus foot deformities, release of the deltoid ligament and PTT, and even transfer of the PTT to the lateral side of the foot, does not result in pathologic valgus foot and ankle position.

A lateralizing or lateral closing wedge calcaneal osteotomy is not always indicated with residual talar tilt after supramalleolar osteotomy; as mentioned, some patients have compensatory hindfoot valgus despite varus talar tilt.[19,51] With the talar tilt passively corrected intraoperatively, we assess the hindfoot position. If the hindfoot is in varus, then a corrective osteotomy is warranted; however, if the heel is in valgus, then a lateralizing calcaneal osteotomy is contraindicated.

Midfoot and first metatarsal osteotomies are indicated when the passive correction of residual talar tilt drives the first ray plantarward. An uncorrected fixed plantarflexion of the medial column of the foot may promote hindfoot varus and recreate the talar tilt. A dorsiflexion osteotomy of the first metatarsal is adequate when the deformity is isolated to the first ray; in some cases, a global pes cavus should be corrected via midfoot dorsiflexion osteotomy and arthrodesis with or without midfoot derotation. In our experience, correction of midfoot cavus is facilitated with plantar fascia release.

Lateral ankle ligament repair/reconstruction and peroneus-to-brevis tendon transfer may be added to further correct residual talar tilt. Occasionally, we also transfer the PTT to the peroneal tendons or to a bony attachment on the lateral foot. Although typically not necessary for a lateral closing wedge supramalleolar osteotomy, Achilles tendon lengthening is often necessary for the medial opening wedge supramalleolar

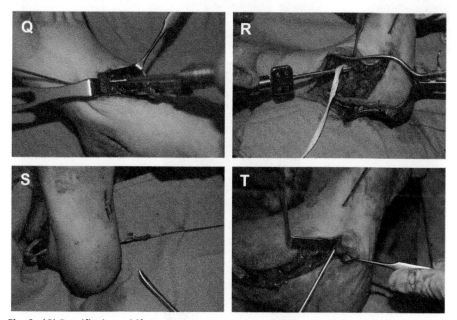

Fig. 6. (Q) Dorsiflexion midfoot osteotomy to correct global cavus deformity. (R, S) Completion of lateral ankle ligament reconstruction using gracilis allograft. (T) PTT anchored to base of the fifth metatarsal.

osteotomy either via gastrocnemius–soleus recession or traditional percutaneous triple hemisection.

Considerations in Treating Both the OLT and Limb Alignment

As we recommended previously in this review, irrespective of varus alignment, the OLT should be treated like an OLT would if there were physiologic ankle alignment. No matter how severe the alignment, an OLT may be managed arthroscopically with debridement and microfracture. An open procedure, with or without medial malleolar osteotomy, typically requires careful planning if it is to be performed in conjunction with realignment, particularly a supramalleolar osteotomy. Osteochondral transfer, autologous chondrocyte transplantation, and structural allograft reconstruction of a section of the medial talar dome often require a medial malleolar osteotomy to allow adequate exposure.[2,8,7,55] Although it is possible to perform both a medial malleolar

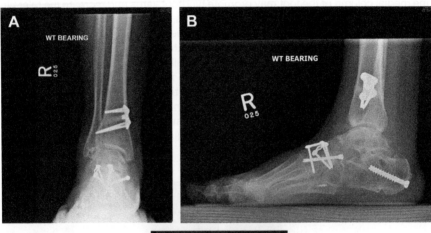

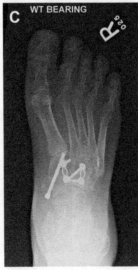

Fig. 7. Two-year follow-up weight-bearing radiographs for same patient in **Figs. 4–6**. (*A*) Ankle mortise. (*B*) Lateral ankle ankle foot. (*C*) Anterior–posterior foot radiograph.

osteotomy and supramalleolar osteotomy simultaneously, in select patients it may be safer to perform these procedures in a carefully planned, staged fashion.

In our hands, a voluminous osteochondral defect distorting the majority of the physiologic anatomy of the medial talar shoulder is best reconstructed with a size-matched medial talar dome structural allograft, replacing one third to one half of the talar dome.[8,10,56] In these cases, we favor an anterior approach, like that performed for total ankle replacement or ankle arthrodesis. Through this anterior approach, simultaneous talar allograft reconstruction and supramalleolar osteotomy is possible, and we typically perform the allograft reconstruction first, followed by the supramalleolar osteotomy. In our experience, foot realignment procedures[50] and

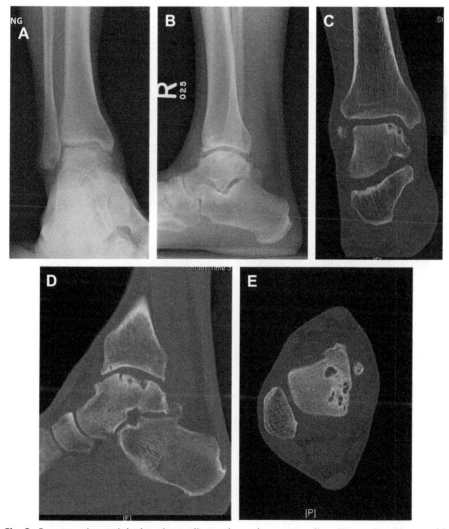

Fig. 8. Preoperative weight-bearing radiographs and corresponding CT scan in a 33 year old patient. (*A*) Ankle mortise demonstrating large talar dome defect and varus talar tilt. (*B*) Lateral ankle. (*C*) Coronal CT. (*D*) Sagittal CT. (*E*) Axial CT.

soft-tissue rebalancing procedures for the foot and ankle[50] performed simultaneous to the surgical management of the OLT and supramalleolar osteotomy may be safely performed through carefully planned surgical approaches.

BIOMECHANICAL STUDIES

In a cadaver model using intra-articular pressure monitoring, Knupp and co-workers[16] demonstrated that a supramalleolar osteotomy indeed shifts center of force and peak pressures laterally. However, with an isolated tibial osteotomy, center of force and peak pressures shifted not only laterally, but also posteriorly. In contrast, when simulating an incongruent deformity by adding a fibular osteotomy, center of force and peak pressures shifted anteromedially. The authors suggested that the effects of supramalleolar osteotomy still need to be fully defined and that more research is needed.

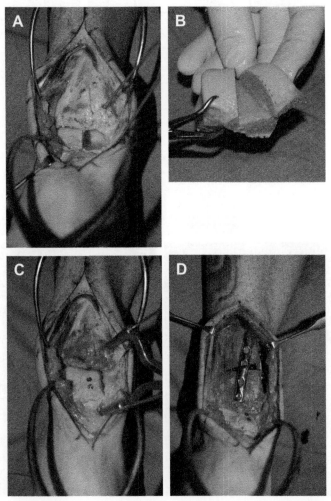

Fig. 9. Intraoperative images of same patient in **Fig. 8.** (*A*) Resection of diseased portion of medial talar dome. (*B*) Talar allograft with carefully separated graft. (*C*) Graft secured to prepared medial talar dome. (*D*) Simultaneous medial opening tibial osteotomy.

We have conducted biomechanical research dedicated to the supramalleolar osteotomy's effect on simulated cartilage defects, including medial talar dome defects.[1] We demonstrated a trend that valgus-producing supramalleolar osteotomies unload the medial cartilage defect, albeit less than we hypothesized and with considerable variability. Our inability to demonstrate statistical significance is perhaps explained by three factors: (1) The ankle–hindfoot couple compensating through the subtalar joint, (2) the concomitant sagittal plane shifts with coronal plane supramalleolar osteotomies observed by Knupp and associates,[15] and/or (3) testing without regard for the influence of in vivo soft-tissue imbalance that may contribute to eccentric peak pressures.

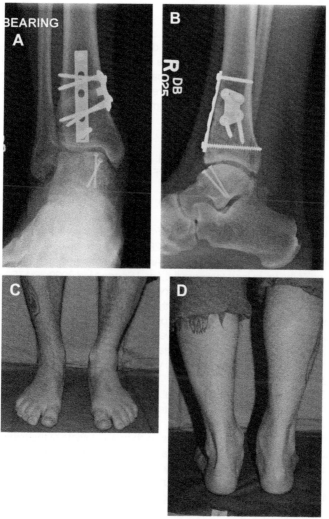

Fig. 10. Three-year follow-up, weight-bearing radiographs and evaluation. (*A*) Anterior–posterior (AP) ankle. (*B*) Lateral ankle. (*C*) AP clinical view. (*D*) Posterior clinical view.

CASE EXAMPLES
Case Example 1

A 38 year-old man presented with severe incongruent tibiotalar varus associated with cavus foot deformity. The patient failed to improve with bracing. We opted to perform a supramalleolar osteotomy in combination with soft-tissue rebalancing and realignment osteotomies of the foot (**Figs. 4–7**).

Case Example 2

A 33 year-old man presented with large, medial talar dome OLT and mild to moderate talar tilt within the ankle mortise. The patient failed nonoperative management and opted for surgical management. Given the size of the uncontained OLT, we performed a fresh structural allograft reconstruction. To correct varus, we added a simultaneous medial opening wedge tibial osteotomy through the same anterior approach (**Figs. 8–10**).

SUMMARY

Considerable recent orthopedic literature is dedicated to either the surgical management of OLTs and correction of varus ankle alignment, but little is published on the combination of these 2 problems. We anticipate that future clinical and biomechanical research will address their simultaneous treatment; until then, we will continue to extrapolate from their independent management.

REFERENCES

1. Wagner EV, Hembree G, Glisson EC, et al. Supramalleolar osteotomies for unloading osteochondral defects of the ankle. In: AOFAS Annual Meeting 2010. National Harbor (MD), July 7–10, 2010.
2. Easley ME, Latt LD, Santangelo JR, et al. Osteochondral lesions of the talus. J Am Acad Orthop Surg 2010;18:616–30.
3. Becher CT, Thermann H. Results of microfracture in the treatment of articular cartilage defects of the talus. Foot Ankle Int 2005;26:583–9.
4. Ferkel RD, Zanotti RM, Komenda GA, et al. Arthroscopic treatment of chronic osteochondral lesions of the talus: long-term results. Am J Sports Med 2008;36:1750–62.
5. Scranton PE Jr, Frey CC, Feder KS. Outcome of osteochondral autograft transplantation for type-V cystic osteochondral lesions of the talus. J Bone Joint Surg Br 2006;88:614–9.
6. Schuman L, Struijs PA, van Dijk CN. Arthroscopic treatment for osteochondral defects of the talus. Results at follow-up at 2 to 11 years. J Bone Joint Surg Br 2002;84(3):364–8.
7. Hangody LK, Kish G, Modis L, et al. Mosaicplasty for the treatment of osteochondritis dessecans of the talus: two to seven year results in 36 patients. Foot Ankle Int 2001;22:552–8.
8. Adams SB Jr, Viens NA, Easley ME, et al. Midterm results of osteochondral lesions of the talar shoulder treated with fresh osteochondral allograft transplantation. J Bone Joint Surg Am 2011;93:648–54.
9. Gross AE, Agnidis Z, Hutchinson CR. Osteochondral defects of the talus treated with fresh osteochondral allograft transplantation. Foot Ankle Int 2001;22:385–91.
10. Raikin SM. Fresh osteochondral allografts for large-volume cystic osteochondral defects of the talus. J Bone Joint Sur Am 2009;91:2818–26.
11. Kono M, Takao M, Naito K, et al. Retrograde drilling for osteochondral lesions of the talar dome. Am J Sports Med 2006;34:1450–6.
12. Robinson DE, Winson IG, Harries WJ, et al. Arthroscopic treatment of osteochondral lesions of the talus. J Bone Joint Surg Br 2003;85:989–93.

13. Savva N, Jabur M, Davies M, et al. Osteochondral lesions of the talus: results of repeat arthroscopic debridement. Foot Ankle Int 2007;28(6):669–73.
14. Harstall R, Lehmann O, Krause F, et al. Supramalleolar lateral closing wedge osteotomy for the treatment of varus ankle arthrosis. Foot Ankle Int 2007;28:542–8.
15. Horn DM, Fragomen AT, Rozbruch SR. Supramalleolar osteotomy using circular external fixation with six-axis deformity correction of the distal tibia. Foot Ankle Int 2011;32:986–93.
16. Knupp M, Stufkens SA, van Bergen CJ, et al. Effect of supramalleolar varus and valgus deformities on the tibiotalar joint: a cadaveric study. Foot Ankle Int 2011;32:609–15.
17. Knupp M, Stufkens SAS, Bolliger L, et al. Classification and treatment of supramalleolar deformities. Foot Ankle Int 2011;32:1023–42.
18. Lee HB. Ligament reconstruction and calcaneal osteotomy for osteoarthritis of the ankle. Foot Ankle Int 2009;30:475–80.
19. Lee WC, Moon JS, Lee K, et al. Indications for supramalleolar osteotomy in patients with ankle osteoarthritis and varus deformity. J Bone Joint Surg Am 2011;93:1243–8.
20. Mann HAM, Myerson MS, Filippi J. Results of medial opening wedge supramalleolar osteotomy (plafond plasty) for the treatment of intraticular varus ankle arthritis and ankle instability. In: 26th Annual Summer Meeting of the American Orthopaedic Foot and Ankle Society 2010. National Harbor (MD), July 7–10, 2010.
21. Pagenstert G, Knupp M, Valderrabana V, et al. Realignment surgery for valgus ankle osteoarthritis. Oper Orthop Traumatol 2009;21:77–87.
22. Pagenstert GI, Hintermann B, Barg A, et al. Realignment surgery as alternative treatment of varus and valgus ankle arthritis. Clin Orthop Relat Res 2007;462:156–68.
23. Takakura Y, Takaoka T, Tanaka Y, et al. Results of opening-wedge osteotomy for the treatment of a post-traumatic varus deformity of the ankle. J Bone Joint Surg Am 1998;80:213–8.
24. Takakura Y, Tanaka Y, Kumai T, et al. Low tibial osteotomy for osteoarthritis of the ankle. Results of a new operation in 18 patients. J Bone Joint Surg Br 1995;77:50–4.
25. Tanaka Y, Takakura Y, Hayashi K, et al. Low tibial osteotomy for varus-type osteoarthritis of the ankle. J Bone Joint Surg Br 2006;88:909–13.
26. Stamatis ED, Cooper PS, Myerson MS. Supramalleolar osteotomy for the treatment of distal tibial angular deformities and arthritis of the ankle joint. Foot Ankle Int 2003;24:754–64.
27. Knupp M, Pagenstert GI, Barg A, et al. SPECT-CT compared with conventional imaging modalities for the assessment of the varus and valgus malaligned hindfoot. J Orthop Res 2009;27:1461–6.
28. Tarr RR, Resnick CT, Wagner KS, et al. Changes in tibiotalar joint contact areas following experimentally induced tibial angular deformities. Clin Orthop Relat Res 1985;199:72–80.
29. Caputo AM, Lee JY, Spritzer CE, et al. In vivo kinematics of the tibiotalar joint after lateral ankle instability. Am J Sports Med 2009;37:2241–8.
30. Komenda GA, Ferkel RD. Arthroscopic findings associated with the unstable ankle. Foot Ankle Int 1999;20:708–13.
31. Bischof JE, Spritzer CE, Caputo AM, et al. In vivo cartilage contact strains in patients with lateral ankle instability. J Biomech 2010;43:2561–6.
32. McKinley TO, Tochigi Y, Rudert MJ, et al. The effect of incongruity and instability on contact stress directional gradients in human cadaveric ankles. Osteoarthritis Cartilage 2008;16:1363–9.
33. Eger WS, Schumacher BL, Mollenhauer J, et al. Human knee and ankle cartilage explants: catabolic differences. J Orthop Res 2002;20:526–34.

34. van Dijk CN, Reilingh ML, Zengerink M, et al. Osteochondral defects in the ankle: why painful? Knee Surg Sports Traumatol Arthrosc 2010;18:570–80.
35. Krause FG, Sutter D, Waehnert D, et al. Ankle joint pressure changes in a pes cavovarus model after lateralizing calcaneal osteotomies. Foot Ankle Int 2010;31:741–6.
36. Sterett WI, Steadman JR, Huang MJ, et al. Chondral resurfacing and high tibial osteotomy in the varus knee: survivorship analysis. Am J Sports Med 2010;38:1420–4.
37. Mina C, Garrett WE Jr, Pietrobon R, et al. High tibial osteotomy for unloading osteochondral defects in the medial compartment of the knee. Am J Sports Med 2008;36:949–55.
38. Bauer S, Khan RJ, Ebert JR, et al. Knee joint preservation with combined neutralising High Tibial Osteotomy (HTO) and Matrix-induced Autologous Chondrocyte Implantation (MACI) in younger patients with medial knee osteoarthritis: a case series with prospective clinical and MRI follow-up over 5years. The Knee 2011. [Epub ahead of print].
39. Leardini A, Stagni R, O'Connor J. Mobility of the subtalar joint in the intact ankle complex. J Biomech 2001;34:805–9.
40. Treppo S, Koepp H, Quan EC, et al. Comparison of biomechanical and biochemical properties of cartilage from human knee and ankle pairs. J Orthop Res 2000;18:739–48.
41. Fetter NL, Leddy HA, Guilak F, et al. Composition and transport properties of human ankle and knee cartilage. J Orthop Res 2006;24:211–9.
42. Ferkel RD, Sgaglione N. Arthroscopic treatment of osteochondral lesions of the talus: long-term results. Orthopaedic Transactions 1990;14:172.
43. Pritsch M, Horoshovski H, Farine I. Arthroscopic treatment of osteochondral lesions of the talus. J Bone Joint Surg Am 1986;68:862–5.
44. Schneider TE, Karaikudi S. Matrix-induced autologous chondrocyte implantation (MACI) grafting for osteochondral lesions of the talus. Foot Ankle Int 2009;30:810–4.
45. Lee KB, Bai LB, Chung JY, et al. Arthroscopic microfracture for osteochondral lesions of the talus. Knee Surg Sports Traumatol Arthrosc 2010;18:247–53.
46. Choi WJ, Park KK, Kim BS, et al. Osteochondral lesions of the talus: is there a critical size for poor outcome? Am J Sports Med 2009;37:1974–80.
47. Han SH, Lee JW, Lee DY, et al. Radiographic changes and clinical results of osteochondral defects of the talus with and without subchondral cysts. Foot Ankle Int 2006;27:1109–14.
48. Taranow WS, Bisignani GA, Towers JD, et al. Retrograde drilling of osteochondral lesions of the medial talar dome. Foot Ankle Int 1999;20:474–80.
49. Mandelbaum BR, Gerhardt MB, Peterson L. Autologous chondrocyte implantation of the talus. Arthroscopy 2003;19(Suppl 1):129–37.
50. Younger AS, Hansen ST Jr. Adult Cavovarus foot. J Am Acad Orthop Surg 2005;13: 302–15.
51. Hayashi K, Tanaka Y, Kumai T, et al. Correlation of compensatory alignment of the subtalar joint to the progression of primary osteoarthritis of the ankle. Foot Ankle Int 2008;29:400–6.
52. Saltzman CL eL-Khoury GY. The hindfoot alignment view. Foot Ankle Int 1995;16: 572–6.
53. Stamatis ED, Myerson MS. Supramalleolar osteotomy: indications and technique. Foot Ankle Clin 2003;8:317–33.
54. Lee KB, Cho YJ. Oblique supramalleolar opening wedge osteotomy without fibular osteotomy for varus deformity of the ankle. Foot Ankle Int 2009;30:565–7.
55. Garras DN, Santangelo JA, Wang DW, et al. A quantitative comparison of surgical approaches for posterolateral osteochondral lesions of the talus. Foot Ankle Int 2008;29:415–20.
56. Raikin, S.M., Stage VI: massive osteochondral defects of the talus. Foot Ankle Clin 2004;9:737–44.

Hindfoot Varus and Neurologic Disorders

Fabian G. Krause, MD[a],*, Lukas D. Iselin, MD[b]

KEYWORDS

- Cavovarus • Charcot-Marie-Tooth disease • Hindfoot varus
- Neurologic disorder • Management

A hindfoot varus often results from muscular imbalance that can be of neurologic, traumatic, congenital, or idiopathic origin. A neurogenic hindfoot varus rarely occurs in isolation and is typically part of a more complex deformity, that is, the cavovarus deformity. Two thirds of adults with symptomatic cavovarus deformity have an underlying neurologic disease, most commonly Charcot-Marie-Tooth (CMT) disease.[1] For successful management, several distinct characteristics of the neurogenic hindfoot varus as opposed to other origins need to be anticipated. This article reviews and updates the etiology, characteristics, and management of the hindfoot varus originating from neurologic disorders.

ETIOLOGY

Many patients present to the orthopedic surgeon with the neurologic disorder already established. A full neurogenic workup is warranted for undiagnosed patients before surgical treatment. CMT is by far the most common underlying neurologic disease causing a hindfoot varus as part of the cavovarus deformity.

CMT Disease

The hereditary motor sensory neuropathy, CMT disease, is by far the most common cause of a cavovarus deformity thought to result from an abnormality of myelination. The disease is an autosomal-dominant hypertrophic neuropathy that clinically occurs in the first or second decade of life.

The musculature innervated by the tibialis nerve fails first. The intrinsics, tibialis anterior, and peroneus brevis are weakened, whereas peroneus longus and extensor hallucis longus are thought to be selectively spared.[2] With rising dysfunction of the

The authors have nothing to disclose.
[a] Department of Orthopaedic Surgery, Inselspital, University of Berne, Freiburgstrasse, 3010 Berne, Switzerland
[b] Royal Adelaide Hospital, Orthopaedic and Trauma Service, North Terrace, Adelaide, SA 5000, Australia
* Corresponding author.
E-mail address: fabian.krause@insel.ch

Foot Ankle Clin N Am 17 (2012) 39–56
doi:10.1016/j.fcl.2011.11.004
1083-7515/12/$ – see front matter © 2012 Elsevier Inc. All rights reserved.

intrinsics, the muscular imbalance of weak anterior tibialis dorsiflexion and strong peroneus longus plantarflexion acting on the medial midfoot initializes the cavovarus deformity.[3] Once the plantarflexion of the medial forefoot, particularly of the first ray, has set in, the strong tibialis posterior induces a forefoot-driven hindfoot varus. This imbalance is caused by the weakened peroneus brevis that serves as the tibialis posterior antagonist in then passively balancing the hindfoot. The hindfoot varus position is also aggravated by direct pull of the tibialis posterior, and with the rising varus position the Achilles tendon contributes to hindfoot varus. Usually hindfoot varus contractures set in later on.[3]

The weakness of tibialis-innervated intrinsic also lead to a claw toe deformity. With the lumbricals not acting to stabilize the metatarsophalangeal (MTP) joints, the unopposed extensor digitorum longus hyperextends the unstable lesser toes at the MTP level, and the flexor digitorum longus and brevis flex the phalanges.[4] The plantarflexed metatarsal heads and plantar fascia shortening add to forefoot equinus.

The cavovarus deformity also occurs in disorders of the spinal cord if the cord or the cauda equina is stretched, deformed or compressed by tumor or structural anomalies, namely, the tethered cord, diastematomyelia.[5]

Cerebral Palsy and Stroke

In childhood, cerebral palsy results from a focal lesion in the brain such as a cyst or hemorrhage. In adults, ischemia and hemorrhage cause strokes. In the resultant hemiplegia, spasticity is seen on 1 side of the body, which in turn may lead to contractures and deformity. Diplegia and total body involvement are less common. In the lower limb, there is typically an equinus or equinovarus deformity due to involvement of the calf muscles.[5] In cerebral palsy, the most common deforming force is the tibialis posterior muscle, whereas in stroke patients the tibialis anterior muscle in conjunction with the triceps surae lead to equinovarus deformity.

Poliomyelitis

The poliovirus affects the anterior horn cells in the spinal cord causing a flaccid lower motor neuron paralysis without any sensory deficit. Wasting and weakness in 1 or more limbs with an equinus or cavovarus deformity after the history of a severe acute illness in early childhood is the typical presentation.[5] Despite continued attempts at universal vaccination, there are new cases every year, and the orthopedic surgeon is occasionally confronted with the sequelae of infection acquired in the past. Generally, orthotic management is efficient, and operative procedures are adjuncts to optimize orthotic fitting.

Myelomeningocele

Myelomeningocele is a congenital malformation of the central nervous system resulting in dysplasia of the vertebral elements and the spinal cord. The most common congenital foot deformity in patients with myelomeningocele is talipes equinovarus (clubfoot), followed by vertical talus, and equinovalgus or -varus deformity.

BIOMECHANICS OF HINDFOOT VARUS

The fixed hindfoot varus is associated with changes in the biomechanics. In the cavovarus deformity, the plantarflexed medial forefoot drives the forefoot into adductus position, the talus into a relative dorsiflexion position within the ankle mortise, and the hindfoot into a varus position. A substantial anteromedial shift of the joint contact pressure has been reported, which in the long term may cause anteromedial ankle arthritis.[6] However, no significant correlation of the (radiographic) deformity's extent or duration and the onset or progression of ankle arthritis has been revealed. Restricted ankle dorsiflexion and discomfort are provoked by an anteromedial ankle impingement.

Moreover, the hindfoot varus leads to a narrowing of the talocalcaneal angle that in turn moves the navicular to a position superior to the cuboid instead of medial to it.[4] The function of the Chopart joint is thereby impaired, and during gait the foot remains locked in hindfoot inversion and forefoot varus throughout the stance phase. The resulting diminished stress distribution may provoke metatarsalgia, fifth ray overload, and lateral hindfoot instability; the locked hindfoot varus likely also contributes to ankle arthritis due to impaired shock absorption at heel strike.

Presentation

Patients with moderate to severe hindfoot varus typically have a significant degree of disability related to their foot shape. Pain and hindfoot instability in conjunction with rising difficulties fitting into shoes motivate these patients to seek medical attention. In the beginning, patients usually complain of discomfort located at the lateral border of foot, metatarsalgia, and recurrent supination sprains. Documenting the frequency of the true chronic hindfoot instability versus sprain apprehension alone is important. Later, patients also report restricted ankle dorsiflexion and discomfort owing to anterior ankle impingement or anteromedial ankle arthritis.

These complaints may be accompanied by progressive symptoms associated with the underlying neurologic disease. Frequent stumbling in running sports after a short period of time may be due to weak ankle dorsiflexors, followed by a complete dropfoot later.

Physical Examination

Meticulous physical examination in conjunction with a clear understanding of the underlying neurologic disease is the key to successful management of the neurogenic hindfoot varus. The severity of involvement of the lower extremities in terms of strength and deformity is frequently asymmetric.[3] In addition, the phenotypic expression of, for example CMT disease, may differ substantially even among family members with similar genotypes.

A complete gait analysis, observation of standing posture, and of the ability to walk on the heels and toes, both in and out of their shoe gear, are required. In CMT, it may reveal a combination of dorsiflexion weakness, fixed equinus, and difficulties with proprioception winding up in the characteristic steppage gait. A screening examination of the back, hips, and knees reveals any relevant biomechanical pathologies (ie, scoliosis, leg length differences). Special attention should be paid to the rotational alignment of the limb from the hip down through the knee and into the foot and ankle.

The standing hindfoot alignment as viewed from the back reveals the extent of the hindfoot varus, and in cavovarus feet the so-called "peek-a-boo" sign indicating a forefoot adductus as well as an elevated medial longitudinal arch (**Fig. 1**A).

Internal and external rotation of the tibia by turning the patient's pelvis provides an initial assessment of how flexible the hindfoot is. The Coleman block test further evaluates the flexibility of the heel and the role of a plantarflexed medial forefoot as the driver of the hindfoot varus (**Fig. 1**B). If the heel corrects completely, the hindfoot varus deformity is thought to be forefoot driven, and the implication is that simply taking care of the plantarflexed first ray corrects the deformity. When the hindfoot remains in a varus position, the hindfoot is considered fixed, and a restoration of the hindfoot alignment including bony and soft-tissue procedures is required as well.

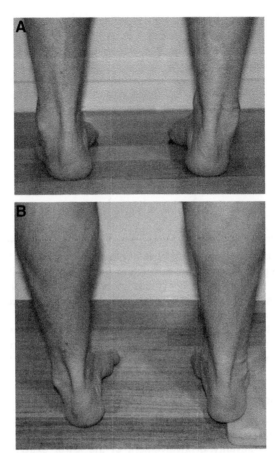

Fig. 1. (*A*) Hindfoot varus alignment in a patient with CMT. Note the "peek-a-boo" sign (visible first ray, no lateral rays), indicating a forefoot adductus and the elevated medial longitudinal arch. (*B*) The Coleman block test defines a flexible deformity as the hindfoot reduces into the physiologic valgus position with the lateral forefoot elevated by the block.

Examination of the foot and ankle is carried out in the seated position. It must record active and passive range of motion for all joints. The Silfverskjøldt test distinguishes between an isolated gastrocnemius contracture and a combined gastrocnemius and soleus contracture. Presence and type of an equinus deformity are assessed. Particular attention is paid to determine whether the ankle rolls normally or functions more as a hinge. Tenderness at the anteromedial ankle suggests arthritis in long-standing deformities. The underlying neuromuscular dysfunction may cause rotatory ankle instability. Documentation of the strength of all muscle groups of the lower extremity is important because it allows an assessment of the progression of the disease over time and helps the surgeon to best understand the options for surgical reconstruction.[3] Discomfort at hindfoot eversion and tenderness along the peroneal tendons imply peroneal tendinopathy. The presence or absence of claw toes, reflexes, sensibility deficiency, and peripheral pulses are noted. Distal migration of the plantar fatpad at the MTP joints in claw toes and the "tripod effect" often cause

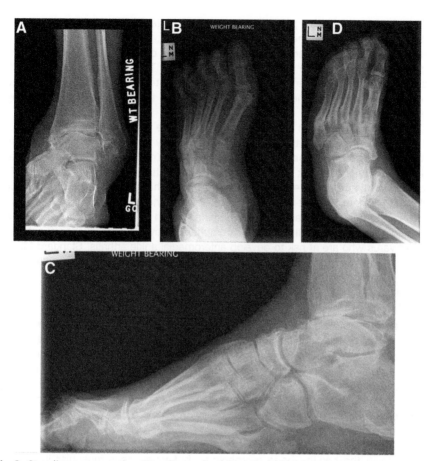

Fig. 2. Standing preoperative AP radiograph of the left ankle (*A*) and AP (*B*), lateral (*C*), and oblique (*D*) radiographs of the foot of a severe left cavovarus foot deformity in a 52-year-old man with CMT disease. Note the varus tilt of the ankle and anteromedial ankle arthritis. Because of the lateral border overload, an old fifth metatarsal fracture is present.

callus formation underneath the first and fifth rays and dorsal ulcerations at the proximal interphalangeal joint level.[7]

At the end of the physical examination, the orthopedic surgeon should have a full understanding of the fore- and hindfoot function and orientation for successful management. If not already made, referral for a neurologic workup is initiated.

Radiographic Examination

At the initial assessment, standing anteroposterior (AP), lateral, and oblique radiographs of the foot and ankle are taken (**Fig. 2**). The characteristics of a hindfoot varus are recorded: A posterior position of the fibula (lateral ankle) and a narrow, almost parallel talocalcaneal angle (AP foot). If the hindfoot varus is part of a cavovarus deformity radiographic additional features are: an increased navicular height, a calcaneal pitch greater than 30°, an increased Hibbs angle (>45°, measured by a line through the axis of the calcaneus and the first metatarsal; in cavovarus feet up to 90°), and an increased angle of Meary (lateral talo–first metatarsal angle; all on the lateral view of the foot), a "flat-topped" talus and an open sinus tarsi area (lateral ankle), and a medially concave talo–first metatarsal angle and fractures of the fifth metatarsal (AP foot). The presence of any arthritic changes (anterior tibial and talar osteophytes, anteromedial ankle joint space narrowing, and osteochondral lesions) is noted and the overall bone morphology should be considered.

Computed tomographic (CT) examination with the foot supported in the typical 90° position with sagittal and coronal reformats may unmask occult degenerative joint disease and tarsal coalitions, and helps with formulating a preoperative plan. In long-standing hindfoot varus, standard magnetic resonance imaging (MRI) illustrates cartilage degeneration and symptomatic hindfoot arthritis by subchondral enhancement. Biochemical T2* MRI has been shown recently to be effective in detecting and quantifying early cartilage degeneration in cavovarus feet that cannot be visualized with standard MRI or plain radiographs.[8] It may allow identifying patients with hindfoot varus who are at risk to develop anteromedial ankle arthritis. Standard MRI or ultrasonography can also be helpful to establish whether tendons are inflamed or torn.

TREATMENT
General Considerations

Because of the variety of the etiologies and the differences in presentation, treatment decisions must be individualized. For management ambulatory versus nonambulatory status has to be carefully assessed. Nonambulatory patients with severe neurologic disorders and mostly equinovarus feet often require a posterior hindfoot release, flexor tendon lengthening (tibialis posterior, flexor digitorum longus and brevis, Achilles), and potentially a peroneus longus to brevis transfer without any additional bony procedures. A plantigrade hindfoot position allows a better fit of orthoses and wheelchair transfer.

When the hindfoot varus is acquired after skeletal maturity, there usually is little or no change in the healthy bone morphology, but when neuromuscular imbalance begins before maturation of the skeleton, there can be substantial change in morphology.[4] Because altered bone morphology may require bony correction other than normal in the neurogenic hindfoot varus, the orthopedic surgeon has to consider the patient's age at onset of the neurologic disease and review the radiographs carefully.

For management, the nature of the underlying neurologic disorder with regard to the likelihood of muscular dystrophy progression and uni- or bilateral affliction has to be anticipated. For example, CMT is typically a bilateral progressive condition, while the unilateral cavovarus foot owing to an asymmetric spinal cord or peripheral nerve injury is unlikely to progress.[3]

Because moderate or even advanced anteromedial ankle arthritis at the time of surgery will likely lead to inferior outcome after deformity realignment, patients with progressive neurologic diseases may benefit from preventive deformity correction. On the other hand, onset and progression of ankle arthritis in hindfoot varus is almost unpredictable by evaluation of the history, physical examination, and plain radiographs or standard MRI. New imaging techniques—biochemical T2* MRI or SPECT CT—have shown promising results for early detection of cartilage degeneration.[8,9] Although no comparative study has proven any advantages of early versus delayed operative treatment to date, in a neurogenic cavovarus foot with deformity progression and any evidence of ankle arthritis early operative realignment may be indicated to neutralize muscle imbalance, and to prevent onset or progression of secondary joint degeneration.[10]

Nonoperative Treatment

The goal of nonoperative treatment of neurogenic hindfoot varus is to alleviate discomfort and improve function. Unless operative treatment is obviously inevitable, every reasonable effort should be made to succeed in nonoperative treatment before surgery.

Physiotherapy

For many CMT patients, chronic lateral hindfoot instability is their initial presenting clinical concern. It is the hindfoot varus, the relative overpull of the medially inserting tendons and the progressive weakness of the peroneus brevis longus, that place excess stress on the lateral hindfoot structures. Efficacy of physiotherapy with peroneal strengthening and proprioception is questionable in this patient population that has sensory and motor deficits but can be attempted.[3] Physiotherapy should primarily focus on preservation of hindfoot and forefoot motion to keep the deformity flexible.

Foot wear

The high-arched cavovarus foot is difficult to fit into regular shoes. Initial supply may include an off-the-shelf lace-up shoe with extra-deep toe boxes. Lace-up boots offer more room and hindfoot stabilization. However, severe cavovarus deformities and claw toes occasionally require extra-depth and custom-made shoes that enable the insertion of orthoses or ankle–foot orthoses (AFO).

Orthoses

Orthoses are valuable adjuncts to the treatment choices for hindfoot varus. They substantially distribute the reduced weight-bearing area in patients with hindfoot varus. Rigid deformities benefit less likely from orthoses, and patients often complain about discomfort and calluses in the supported areas.

For the common lateral instability in hindfoot varus, a high top boot or an off-the-shelf ankle brace offer external hindfoot stabilization. Lace-up braces are easier to fit inside a shoe or boot, and stabilization of the ankle is equal to plastic upright braces. Medial arch supporting orthoses aggravate preexisting hindfoot varus and therefore hindfoot instability as well.

To prevent problems arising from dropfoot, muscle weakness is frequently treated with a full-length, custom AFO. Orthotic modifications integrated into the AFO provide better comfort, proprioception, and hindfoot stability control than a brace alone. Ankle braces are also essential to avoid any progression of an equinus contracture. If progression occurs anyway, an additional night-splint or even clamshell braces or below-the-knee casts should be applied.

OPERATIVE TREATMENT OF HINDFOOT VARUS ORIGINATING FROM CMT

Next to a plantarflexed medial forefoot and a forefoot adductus, the hindfoot varus is one of the major components in the cavovarus deformity originating from CMT. Next to alleviation of discomfort and improvement of function, the goal of operative treatment is to prevent or halt anteromedial ankle arthritis. The patient should be informed early about these goals, expected outcome, and recovery time after surgery. In the majority of patients with neurogenic cavovarus feet, an appropriate correction of the foot is achieved with soft-tissue release, tendon transfers, and osteotomies.[1,11]

Almost all studies also report a lateral hindfoot ligament repair or reconstruction as part of the correction. It is our experience that, with complete static and dynamic realignment of the deformity, hindfoot stability is achieved even without ligamentous stabilization.

Soft-tissue contractures are released to restore the normal foot shape (plantar fascia release). Tendons contributing to the deformity are transferred to a more functional location strengthening weak muscles (tibialis posterior to the dorsum of the foot). Corrective osteotomies are preferable to arthrodeses of joints with no or mild arthritis, but symptomatic joints with advanced arthritis should be fused. Osteotomies usually offer the same potential of correction but restore motion of the already less flexible cavovarus foot (calcaneal osteotomy instead of a subtalar fusion).

General treatment options should be applied cautiously to specific patients with underlying neurologic disorder because of substantial interindividual phenotypic variability.

Soft-Tissue Release and Tendon Lengthening

Medial and plantar soft-tissue contractures are part of the cavovarus deformity. In severe and rigid deformities with restricted ankle dorsiflexion and a tight posterior capsule, a posteromedial soft-tissue release is mandatory for a full correction. For a tight heel cord, either a gastrocnemius recession or open Achilles lengthening is performed. A gastrocnemius recession may be indicated if the gastrocnemius component of the triceps surae alone is tight (positive Silfverskjöld test). Anterior talar and tibial osteophytes indicating anteromedial ankle arthritis also restrict ankle dorsiflexion, and symptomatic anterior ankle impingement is treated by open or arthroscopic debridement and osteophytectomy (**Fig. 3**). Anterior osteophytes are well illustrated by weight-bearing lateral ankle radiographs. Heel cord lengthening in these cases is not reasonable, because it reduces toe-off power and increases anterior ankle impingement, although it does not improve ankle dorsiflexion.

Aside from an open tenotomy, a percutaneous tenotomy is an option for heel cord lengthening. Achilles overlengthening may provoke calcaneus gait and weak ankle plantarflexion. A lengthening tenotomy or a split tibialis posterior tendon transfer at the same time may be considered when a hindfoot varus is present in the stance phase of gait.[12] If the toes are flexed in the plantigrade foot position, a flexor digitorum longus lengthening is also indicated, and the contracted flexor hallucis tendon may be released at the knot of Henry for a tight first ray. A transfer of the flexor hallucis tendon into a weak or paralyzed peroneus brevis was found to be very efficient.[13]

In severe gastrocnemius contractures, the isolated tendon is completely sectioned (Strayer procedure), whereas in mild contractures only the aponeurosis is sectioned while the muscle fibers are left intact (Baumann procedure).[14,15] After the recession, improved ankle dorsiflexion is assessed with the knee in extension. The value of a gastrocnemius recession in cavovarus realignment still lacks evidence in the literature. If soft-tissue contractures continue to impair ankle dorsiflexion after heel cord lengthening, a posterior ankle and subtalar joint capsule release and a deltoid ligament release at the posterior aspect of the medial malleolus may eliminate restriction.

For a high-arched midfoot, a plantar fascia release in its mid-portion, or in severe cases, an extensive release from the calcaneus with releases of the deep muscles and their tendon sheaths, are suggested.[16,17] Also, a dorsomedial talonavicular capsulotomy of the usually contracted joint adds to correction of the high arch.

Tendon Transfer

The basic requirements for tendon transfer are as follows. Agonists are preferable to antagonists.[16] Joints affected by the tendons transfer should provide reasonable function (range of motion, stability, and no or minor deformity). Because 1 grade of strength is usually lost with the transfer, the transferred muscle should have appropriate strength and excursion. The transferred tendon should be inserted close to the former insertion of the substituted tendon and routed directly without angulation. Insertion should be either directly in bone, or indirectly by using another tendon's weave. Tension should be slight to moderate, approximately half of the tendon's excursion. The tendon's nerve and blood supply should be preserved.[16]

Tendon transfers are divided into "in-phase" versus "out-of-phase" and "swing-phase" versus "stance-phase." In-phase transfers are certainly preferable (**Tables 1** and **2**). As opposed to whole tendon transfer, split transfer is considered less effective but more reliable because it distributes the muscle power more equally and reduces the risk of overcorrection.[18] Conversely, to our knowledge, overcorrection as postoperative complication in an adult neurogenic hindfoot varus has not been reported in the literature. For example, the donor morbidity after tibialis posterior transfer in cavovarus realignment is negligible, because bony and ligamentous architecture prevent arch collapse. Moreover, residual deformity owing to incomplete correction is a common reason for an unsatisfying outcome.

Sole soft-tissue procedures are usually sufficient in the flexible hindfoot varus. If the deformity correction is not completed after extended soft-tissue releases and tendon

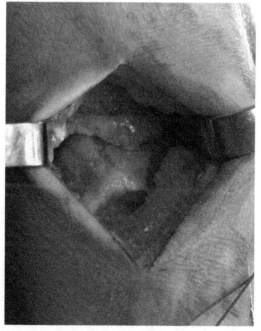

Fig. 3. Left ankle medial arthrotomy of the same patient presented in **Fig. 2**. Note the anterior tibial osteophytes and the anteromedial cartilage erosion on the talus.

Table 1
"In-phase" transfers

Donor	Recipient	Indication	Concomitant Procedure
Swing phase			
Extensor hallucis longus	Tibialis anterior	Clawed first ray, weak dorsiflexion	First ray IP fusion, MTP joint release
Extensor hallucis longus	Peroneus tertius (complete or split)	Weak dorsiflexion with inversion on swing phase	First ray IP fusion, MTP joint release
Extensor digitorum brevis	Extensor digitorum longus stump	Claw toes	IP fusions or excisions, MTP joint releases
Extensor digitorum longus	Peroneus tertius	Clawed lesser toes, weak dorsiflexion	IP fusions or excisions, MTP joint releases
Tibialis anterior—complete or split	Peroneus tertius	Excessive forefoot inversion during swing phase	
Stance phase			
Flexor hallucis longus	Peroneus Brevis	Weak ankle eversion	Calcaneal osteotomy
Flexor hallucis longus	Peroneus Longus	Flexible forefoot varus	Midfoot fusion
Peroneus longus	Peroneus Brevis	Weak ankle eversion	Calcaneal osteotomy
Peroneus brevis	Peroneus longus	Weak ankle eversion and flexible forefoot varus	Calcaneal osteotomy
Tibialis posterior—complete or split	Peroneus brevis	Weak ankle eversion	Calcaneal osteotomy
Tibialis posterior—complete or split	Peroneus longus	Forefoot varus and weak ankle eversion	Calcaneal osteotomy

Abbreviation: IP, interphalangeal.
©2005 American Academy of Orthopaedic Surgeons. (*Reprinted from* the Journal of the American Academy of Orthopaedic Surgeons, Volume 13 (5). pp. 302-315; with permission.)

Table 2
"Out-of-phase" transfer for swing phase deficits

Donor	Recipient	Indication	Concomitant Procedure
Tibialis posterior	Tibialis anterior and/or peroneus tertius	Weak dorsiflexion—lower motor neuron cause	Heel cord lengthening
Peroneus longus	Peroneus tertius	Weak dorsiflexion	Tibialis posterior transfer; heel cord lengthening
Flexor hallucis longus and digitorum longus	Fourth metatarsal through interosseous membrane	Weak dorsiflexion due to stroke	Short flexor release; lengthening of heel cord or tibialis posterior
Flexor digitorum longus	Extensor hood	Intrinsic deformity of toes	IP joint fusion or excision

Abbreviation: IP, interphalangeal.

©2005 American Academy of Orthopaedic Surgeons. (*Reprinted from* the Journal of the American Academy of Orthopaedic Surgeons, Volume 13 (5), pp. 302-315; with permission.)

transfers, the hindfoot varus is obviously at least partially fixed, and osteotomies or arthrodeses are required in addition to fully realign the deformity.

Osteotomy

For realignment of neurogenic cavovarus feet, osteotomies are preferred over arthrodeses whenever possible. For severe single components of the entire deformity, osteotomies are occasionally combined with an arthrodesis or another osteotomy. For example, if a lateralizing calcaneal osteotomy cannot completely correct a severe varus ankle–hindfoot alignment, an additional valgus subtalar arthrodesis or valgus tibial osteotomy may add to the realignment.

Next to hindfoot varus, an internally rotated distal tibia accentuates the varus lever of the Achilles tendon. The resultant internally rotated forefoot contributes towards medial ankle joint overload. CT is useful for the assessment of tibial torsion.[19] A supramalleolar osteotomy or a lateral column shortening then derotates the forefoot, redistributes the elevated ankle pressure, and realigns the hindfoot.

Calcaneal Osteotomies

A lateralizing calcaneal osteotomy predominantly without subtalar fusion is indicated, when the hindfoot does not correct passively to neutral. In cavovarus foot deformities, it realigns the hindfoot varus during heel strike and lateralizes the lever arm of the Achilles tendon during toe-off. The contribution of the Achilles tendon toward the tibialis posterior is thus reduced in favor of the peroneus brevis.

In a recent biomechanical study, realignment of a simulated fixed hindfoot varus by tested common lateralizing calcaneal osteotomies contributed substantially to normalize elevated anteromedial ankle contact stresses in hindfoot varus.[20] In combination with other soft-tissue and bony procedures, calcaneal osteotomies therefore seem to prevent onset or progression of anteromedial ankle joint arthritis in hindfoot varus by correction of the deformity's static components. Although the lateral sliding osteotomy of the calcaneal tuberosity and the Z-shaped laterally closing osteotomy with additional lateralization of the tuberosity (Hintermann)[21] were more effective and should add to normalize ankle joint contact stresses in severe hindfoot varus deformities, the less effective "Italian" L-shaped (Pisani)[22] or Z-shaped (Malerba)[23] laterally closing osteotomies without additional lateralization of the tuberosity, may be considered mild cavovarus deformities. The simple, straight-cut, lateral sliding osteotomy of the calcaneal tuberosity was as effective as the more complex Z-shaped laterally closing osteotomy with additional lateralization of the tuberosity.[20]

The Dwyer closing wedge osteotomy decreases the lever arm of the Achilles tendon.[24] However, complete realignment is achieved in mild deformities only, and a sliding calcaneal osteotomy without excision is usually preferable.[13]

The posterior calcaneal osteotomy with plantar release is applied for realignment of a very high-arched cavovarus foot in conjunction with a weak triceps surae. The tuberosity is displaced posteriorly and superiorly using an oblique osteotomy. The increased calcaneal pitch is reduced, and the lever arm of the weak muscle is improved, but it may impair preexisting anterior ankle impingement.[25]

Particularly in cavovarus deformity with underlying peripheral neuropathy, the peripheral nerves are thickened and symptomatic compression of the tibial nerve is seen after any lateral sliding of the calcaneal tuberosity. In CMT and other patients with peripheral neuropathy, decompression of the medial neurovascular bundle under the flexor retinaculum is advisable.[26]

Lateral Column Shortening

In the majority of neurogenic cavovarus deformities, realignment of the foot on the tibia is achieved after release of the talonavicular joint. After soft tissue releases, the need for lateral column shortening is determined by assessment of the foot position. When the forefoot varus and adductus fail to correct after dorsomedial talonavicular release, a lateral column shortening adds to realignment. It can be performed through the cuboid, the calcaneus, or through the calcaneo-cuboid joint.[16]

Dorsiflexion Osteotomy of the First Ray

Dorsiflexion of the first ray is attained by a dorsal closing osteotomy of the first metatarsal or the medial cuneiform (reversed Cotton osteotomy).

A plantarflexed first ray is common in CMT disease. Indications for a dorsiflexion osteotomy are a symptomatic and plantarflexed first ray with discomfort owing to overload of the first ray, forefoot-driven hindfoot varus (positive Coleman block test), and overloaded lateral border. Usually, the plantarflexed first ray is seen in combination with clawing of the first ray owing to dorsal contracture of the MTP joint capsules and tight extensor tendons. A dorsiflexion arthrodesis through the first tarsometatarsal joint should be considered for hypermobile or arthritic joints, a short first ray, or a strong peroneus longus plantarflexing the first ray. Hallux rigidus and transfer metatarsalgia has been reported for overcorrection with excessive shortening and elevation of the first ray.[27] Dorsiflexion osteotomy of the second and third metatarsals is added when simulated intraoperative weight bearing demonstrates an overload of their heads after first ray dorsiflexion. For an unrestricted elevation of the metatarsals, a release of the plantar fascia may be essential.

To avoid shortening and transfer metatarsalgia by a corrective first tarsometatarsal arthrodesis, very little bone should be removed. A simultaneous Jones transfer and dorsal capsulotomy may be required for release of the first MTP joint.

Midfoot Osteotomy

With the rationale being that the midfoot is the apex of the deformity, midfoot osteotomies for cavovarus realignment are performed by removal of a dorsally or dorsolaterally based wedge-shaped bony segment. The Jahss osteotomy[28] is a truncated wedge osteotomy through the mid tarsal region, whereas the Japas osteotomy[29] is essentially a vertical chevron osteotomy through the mid tarsal region. A simultaneous plantar fascia release facilitates realignment through the osteotomy. Given that high rates of residual opening, malunion, and nonunion at the osteotomy site were reported, most orthopedic surgeons abandoned midfoot osteotomies.[1,30]

Hindfoot Arthrodesis

A corrective subtalar arthrodesis allows additional hindfoot valgus with realignment through the subtalar joint, when the hindfoot varus cannot be fully corrected by osteotomies. It can be done in addition to the calcaneal osteotomy or as an independent procedure.

Occasionally, in severe and rigid neurogenic hindfoot varus or equinovarus deformity, a double or triple arthrodesis is required to position the foot appropriately beneath the ankle. Some authors concluded in their studies that for definite correction of neurogenic hindfoot varus a triple arthrodesis is a precondition for good outcome in children and adolescents.[31,32] Even after triple arthrodesis,

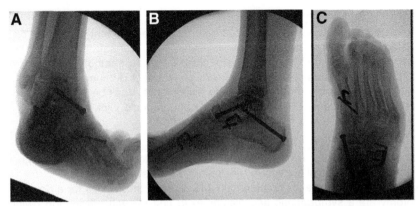

Fig. 4. (*A–C*) Intraoperative radiographs of the same patient presented in **Fig. 2**. A corrective triple arthrodesis for the arthritic talonavicular and subtalar joints and a dorsiflexion osteotomy of the first ray were performed. No further soft-tissue procedure was required for realignment. (*Courtesy of* Dr G. Dragopoulos, Adelaide.)

muscular imbalance might cause recurrence of hindfoot varus through the ankle and need to be balanced.

Although deformity correction is fairly reliable, the downsides of triple arthrodeses include loss of motion and, particularly in younger patients with normal life span, adjacent joint arthritis. Accordingly, variable outcomes and a high incidence of ankle and midfoot arthritis frequently requiring ankle fusions are reported in long-term follow-up studies after triple arthrodesis for neurogenic hindfoot varus.[33,34] However, occasionally arthritic hindfoot joints may obligate an arthrodesis (**Fig. 4**). The original and modified Lambrinudi procedure that regained more interest within the last years is a modification of the triple arthrodesis and is performed when severe anterior muscle weakness and rigid dropfoot are present.[35,36]

Currently, joint-preserving bony procedures in association with soft-tissue procedures to realign the hindfoot varus are considered preferable to hindfoot arthrodeses. Triple arthrodesis should be regarded as a salvage procedure, and the number of joints fused to achieve the desired correction should be limited.

Clawtoe Reconstruction

Flexible or rigid clawtoes are commonly seen in conjunction with neurogenic hindfoot varus; dynamic clawtoes may resolve after realignment of the hindfoot deformity. A flexor-to-extensor tendon transfer with either the Girdlestone-Taylor procedure is recommended for dynamic clawing with flexible deformity.[16] Proximal interphalangeal joint arthrodeses have a similar effect on the long flexor tendons, require less dissection, and are preferable for the fixed clawtoe deformity. At the same time, a Jones transfer or extensor tendon (modified Hibbs) transfer to the lateral border of the foot may be indicated.

TREATMENT OF HINDFOOT VARUS ORIGINATING FROM NEUROLOGIC DISEASE OTHER THAN CMT

Botulinum toxin, which interrupts motor endplate function, allows temporary tone reduction in spasticity. Spasticity may also be reduced by selective destruction of the dorsal spinal roots (selective dorsal rhizotomy—a procedure that has not found much favor in the United Kingdom) or by continuous intrathecal infusion of baclofen, a tone-reducing drug.[5] Surgery should be avoided in younger patients because it may interfere with muscle growth.

Out-of-phase tendon transfers are occasionally used in younger patients with lower motor neuron pathology (ie, tibialis posterior to tibialis anterior transfer). Tibialis anterior and posterior split tendon transfers are applied in children with cerebral palsy. Increased dorsiflexion strength is achieved with an anterior transfer of the long toe flexors in patients with hemiplegia.[37]

In poliomyelitis, it has to be considered that surgery can never increase muscle power but may contribute to further weakness. Nevertheless, a functioning tibialis posterior tendon transfer through the interosseous membrane onto the dorsum of the foot to counteract an equinovarus deformity may be indicated. However, surgical effort is usually concentrated on simple bony procedures to correct fixed deformities and enable use of appropriate orthoses. The equinus and cavovarus deformities in poliomyelitis may require either hindfoot fusions or midfoot osteotomies.[5] Good results for rotational tibial osteotomies that also externally rotate the foot in patients with polio and other neurologic disorders have been reported.[38] The osteotomy decreases the varus lever of the Achilles' tendon at the subtalar joint and unlocks the subtalar joint.

In the younger child with hemiplegia and a flexible equinovarus deformity, a sole transfer of the tibialis posterior tendon has been advocated. In the rigid deformity, the orthopedic surgeon may also consider a lateralizing calcaneal osteotomy, a closing wedge osteotomy of the cuboid and opening wedge osteotomy of the cuneiform, a medial hindfoot release, and a tibialis posterior tendon lengthening with split transfer to the peroneus brevis tendon. Improved dorsiflexion strength is achieved with an anterior split transfer of the long toe flexors.[37]

In stroke patients, it is the tibialis posterior overpull that supinates the hindfoot and midfoot into a varus position and, in conjunction with the triceps surae, results the equinovarus posture. Mild deformities respond well to orthotics (ie, AFO), whereas more rigid deformities with tight tibialis posterior tendons benefit from a tibialis posterior tendon transfer or lengthening in conjunction with heel cord lengthening.[17] For a dropfoot in stroke patients, an anterior transfer of the flexor digitorum longus and flexor hallucis longus may be used.[39]

Extensive releases may expose underlying weakness of the involved muscles and impair appropriate rehabilitation in older children. Excessive lengthening of the heel cord may wind up in an aggravated cavovarus deformity with anterior ankle impingement, in a calcaneus gait with weak plantarflexion and poor gait progression, and in a recruitment of the quadriceps costing the patient more energy during gait.[40] The failed release of tight long toe flexors leads to painful calluses underneath claw toes.[41] Although appropriate releases and tendon transfers may create neutral foot realignment and improve or prevent bracing, walking ability is limited by age at surgery and degree of paralysis.[39]

Talipes equinovarus in myelomeningocele do by majority come to surgery; however, early serial casting should be tried initially. Early surgery includes complete subtalar release and resection of deformity producing tendons. Later, triple arthrodesis or talectomy may be considered for correction.

Outcomes

Few published studies report generally good outcomes for hindfoot varus treatment in patients with neurologic disorders. Because of the low number of patients treated, the variability among patients, and their treatment, only sparse conclusions from these studies can be drawn. Patients with no to minimal preoperative ankle arthritis seem to have higher clinical scores after cavovarus realignment and increased satisfaction than those with more advanced arthritis.[40] Patients with neuropathy tend to suffer from more postoperative pain and impairment of daily activities than idiopathic patients after hindfoot varus correction. Even after complete correction, the muscle weakness around the hindfoot likely prevents improvement of balance.

It is our experience that even the long-term outcomes in patients with cavovarus deformity and mild to moderate anteromedial ankle arthritis are generally good when full alignment has been achieved, without significant differences between idiopathic and neurogenic etiologies for hindfoot varus. Particularly when the talus varus tilt has been corrected, there is no ankle arthritis progression over the years, whereas to achieve neutral ankle alignment occasionally requires fibula shortening osteotomy in addition. Even without lateral ligament repair or reconstruction, patients with preoperative lateral hindfoot instability all gained sufficient stability with static and dynamic realignment.

SUMMARY

Muscle imbalance from numerous underlying neurologic disorders can cause dynamic and static hindfoot varus deformity. Most etiologies are congenital, and therefore affect bone morphology and the shape of the foot during growth. Weak and strong muscle groups, bone deformity, and soft-tissue contractures have to be carefully assessed and considered for successful management. Because of the variety of the etiologies and the differences in presentation, treatment decisions in varus hindfoot caused by neurologic disorders must be individualized. Deformity correction includes release of soft tissue contractures, osteotomies and arthrodeses, and tenotomies or tendon transfers to balance muscle strength and prevent recurrence. To decrease elevated anteromedial ankle joint contact stress and provide lateral hindfoot stability during the entire gait cycle, the goal of static and dynamic hindfoot varus realignment is to fully correct all components of the deformity, but particularly the varus tilt of the talus.

REFERENCES

1. Alexander IJ, Johnson KA. Assessment and management of pes cavus in Charcot-Marie-Tooth disease. Clin Orthop 1989;246:273–81.
2. Mann RA, Missirian J. Pathophysiology of Charcot-Marie-Tooth disease. Clin Orthop Rel Res 1988;234:221–8.
3. Beals TC, Nickisch F. Charcot-Marie-Tooth disease and the cavovarus foot. Foot Ankle Clin North Am 2008;13:259–74.
4. Aminian A, Sangeorzan BJ. The anatomy of cavus foot deformity. Foot Ankle Clin North Am 2008;13:191–8.
5. Paterson JM. Neuromuscular conditions of childhood. Surgery 29;4:191–6.
6. Krause F, Windolf M, Schwieger K, et al. Ankle joint pressure in pes cavovarus. J Bone Joint Surg Br 2007;89-B:1660–1665.
7. Kroon M, Faber WM, Van der Linden M. Joint preservation surgery for correction of flexible pes cavovarus in adults. Foot Ankle Int 2010;31:24–9.
8. Krause FG, Klammer G, Benneker LM, et al. Biochemical T2* MR quantification of ankle arthrosis in pes cavovarus. J Orthop Res 2010;28:1562–8.
9. Pagenstert G, Barg A, Leumann A, et al. SPECT-CT imaging in degenerative joint disease of the foot and ankle. 2009 J Bone Joint Surg Br 2010;91:1191–6.
10. Younger ASE, Hansen ST. Adult cavovarus foot. J Am Acad Orthop Surg 2005;13:302–15.

11. Jahss MH. Evaluation of the cavus foot for orthopaedic treatment. Clin Orthop Rel Res 1983;181:52–63.
12. Kagaya H, Yamada S, Nagasawa T, et al. Split posterior tibial tendon transfer for varus deformity of hindfoot. Clin Orthop 1996;323:254–60.
13. Hansen ST Jr. Functional reconstruction of the foot and ankle. Philadelphia: Lippincott Williams & Wilkins; 2000.
14. Baumann JU, Koch HG. Ventrale aponeurotische Verlängerung des Musculus gastrocnemius. Operat Orthop Traumatol 1989;1:254–248.
15. Strayer LM Jr. Recession of the gastrocnemius: an operation to relieve spastic contracture of the calf muscles. J Bone Joint Surg Am 1950;32:671–6.
16. Ingram AJ. Paralytic disorders. In: Crenshaw AH, editor. Campbell's orthopaedics. 7th edition. St. Louis: Mosby; 1987. p. 2925–3061.
17. Sherman FC, Westin GW. Plantar release in the correction of deformities of the foot in childhood. J Bone Joint Surg Am 1981;63:1382–9.
18. Vlachou M, Dimitriadis D. Split tendon transfers for the correction of spastic foot deformity: a case series study. J Foot Ankle Res 2010;3:28–39.
19. Liggio FJ, Kruse R. Split tibial posterior transfer with concomitant distal tibia derotational osteotomy in children with cerebral palsy. J Pediatr Orthop 2001;21: 95–101.
20. Krause FG, Sutter D, Waehnert D, et al. Ankle joint pressure changes in a pes cavovarus model after lateralizing calcaneal osteotomies. Foot Ankle Int 2010;31: 741–6.
21. Knupp M, Horisberger M, Hintermann B. A new Z-shaped calcaneal osteotomy for 3-plane correction of severe deformity of the hindfoot. Tech Foot Ankle Surg 2008; 7:90–5.
22. Pisani G. Osteotomia sottotalamica di sottrazione laterale. In: Trattato di chirurgia del piede. Torino (Italy): Edizioni Minerva Medica S.p.A.; 1990:287–8.
23. Malerba F, De Marchi F. Calcaneal osteotomies. Foot Ankle Clin 2005;10:523–40.
24. Dwyer FC. The present status of the problem of pes cavus. Clin Orthop 1975;106: 254–75.
25. Mitchell GP. Posterior displacement osteotomy of the calcaneus. J Bone Joint Surg Br 1977;59:233–5.
26. Krause FG, Pohl MJ, Penner MJ, et al. Tibial nerve palsy associated with lateralizing calcaneal osteotomy: case reviews and technical tip. Foot Ankle Int 2009;30:258–61.
27. Breusch SJ, Wenz W, Doederlein L. Function after correction of a clawed great toe by a modified Robert Jones transfer. J Bone Joint Surg Br 2000;82:250–4.
28. Jahss MH. Tarsometatarsal truncated wedge arthrodesis for pes cavus and equinovarus deformity of the forepart of the foot. J Bone Joint Surg Am 1980;62:713–22.
29. Japas LM. Surgical treatment of pes cavus by tarsal v-osteotomy. J Bone Joint Surg Am 1968;50:927–44.
30. Watanabe RS. Metatarsal osteotomy for the cavus foot. Clin Orthop 1990;252: 217–30.
31. Jacobs JE, Carr CR. Progressive muscular atrophy of the peroneal type (Charcot-Marie-Tooth disease). Orthopaedic management and end-result study. J Bone Joint Surg Am 1950;32:27–38.
32. Levitt RL, Cooke AJ, Graland JJ. The role of foot surgery in progressive neuromuscular disorders in children. J Bone Joint Surg Am 1973;55:1396–410.
33. Wetmore RS, Drennan JC. Long-term results of triple arthrodesis in Charcot-Marie-Tooth disease. J Bone Joint Surg Am 1989;71:417–22.

34. Saltzmann CL, Fehrle MJ, Cooper RR, et al. Triple arthrodesis: twenty-five and forty-four average follow-up of the same patients. J Bone Joint Surg Am 1999;81: 1391–402.

35. Lambrinudi C. New operation of drop-foot. Br J Surg 1927;15:193–200.

36. Elsner A, Barg A, Stufkens S, et al. Modified Lambrinudi arthrodesis with additional posterior tibial tendon transfer in adult drop foot. Oper Orthop Traumatol 2011;23: 121–30.

37. Morita S, Yamamoto H, Furuya K. Anterior transfer of the toe flexors for equinovarus deformity due to hemiplegia. J Bone Joint Surg Br 1994;76:447–9.

38. McNichol D, Leong JC, Hsu LC. Supramalleolar derotation osteotomy for lateral tibial torsion and associated equinovarus deformity of the foot. J Bone Joint Surg Br 1983;65:166–70.

39. Yamamoto H, Okumura S, Morita S, et al. Surgical correction of foot deformities after stroke. Clin Orthop 1992;282:213–8.

40. Johnson WL, Lester EL. Transposition of the posterior tibial tendon. Clin Orthop 1989;245:223–7.

41. Keenan MA, Gorai AP, Smith CW, et al. Intrinsic toe flexors deformity following correction of spastic equinovarus in adults. Foot Ankle, 1987;7:333–7.

The Varus Ankle and Instability

Georg Klammer, MD, Emanuel Benninger, MD,
Norman Espinosa, MD*

KEYWORDS

• Varus • Ankle • Instability • Treatment

Hindfoot varus has been recognized as an anatomic risk factor that promotes chronic lateral ankle instability.[1–3] Hindfoot varus is present in 8% of patients with ankle instability, and with 28% it is the most commonly found condition in patients with persisting pain or recurrent instability after lateral ankle ligament reconstruction.[4] Varus malalignment may occur isolated at a single structural level (eg, supramalleolar) or as part of a complex deformity with multiple structures involved (eg, cavovarus deformity). In order to select the optimal treatment strategy, a thorough understanding of the static and dynamic causes of deformity and their biomechanical effects is mandatory.

BIOMECHANICS IN THE VARUS ANKLE

Abnormalities in the frontal, sagittal, and/or transversal plane of the hindfoot lead to asymmetric force distributions across the joints.[5] As such, it is the nature of a varus hindfoot that medial joint areas become overloaded, bearing the potential for premature degeneration of the cartilage.[6,7] However, compared with a valgus ankle, progression of osteoarthritis in a varus ankle is slow. The reason for this slow progression has been found in a stronger medial bone support, which theoretically could be protective and delay arthritic changes.[8,9] In addition, kinematics at the hindfoot are altered as a result of a misdirected pulling vector of the Achilles tendon. At heel strike, the varus hindfoot provokes an inversion moment exerted by the Achilles tendon. Thus, the strain on the lateral structures of the ankle is increased and the ligaments are exposed to a higher failure risk. Recurrent ankle sprain in patients with varus malalignment of the hindfoot is a frequent finding.[10] Up to 30% of patients who have been operated on for recurrent ankle instability reveal some kind of hindfoot varus that has not been detected at the initial workup.[4] Lateral instability itself is the second most common cause of posttraumatic osteoarthritis of the ankle.[11] The combination of mechanical and functional instability at the hindfoot—as typically present in varus

The authors have nothing to disclose.

Foot and Ankle Surgery, Department of Orthopaedics, University of Zurich, Balgrist, Forchstrasse 340, 8008 Zurich, Switzerland
* Corresponding author.
E-mail address: norman.espinosa@balgrist.ch

Table 1 Causes of simple hindfoot varus malalignment	
Source of Hindfoot Varus	Clinical Example
- Knee	Medial osteoarthritis
- Lower leg	Malunited tibial fracture
- Supramalleolar	Malunited pilon fracture
Tibiotalocalcaneal varus	
- Ankle joint	Chronic instability with varus osteoarthritis
- Talocalcaneal	Tarsal coalition
- Calcaneal	Malunited calcaneal fracture

deformities—promotes the development of ankle osteoarthritis.[12–15] Based on these facts, varus malalignment of the hindfoot must be recognized and addressed when treating instability of the ankle and subtalar joint.[16]

ANATOMIC CHARACTERISTICS OF SIMPLE AND COMPLEX VARUS HINDFOOT DEFORMITY
Simple Hindfoot Varus Malalignment

In isolated hindfoot varus deformities, malalignment is the result of an anatomic aberration at a single level either below at or above the ankle joint (**Table 1**).[17–19] The lever arm of the Achilles tendon is increased and its pulling vector medialized. Therefore, the inversion moment at the hindfoot is increased.[20] In case of a fixed varus deformity at the subtalar joint, the situation is worse because compensatory movement in inversion and eversion takes place solely at the ankle.[21] Thus, the susceptibility to an ankle sprain or chronic ankle instability is high. Over time, hindfoot varus may result in additional midfoot and forefoot malalignment, transforming a simple and isolated varus deformity into a complex one.

Complex Varus Deformities

Regarding complex deformities, the hindfoot varus is one element of a multitude of structures contributing to the malalignment of the foot and ankle. The most common type of such a deformity is the cavovarus foot.[22] A synopsis of causes leading to cavovarus deformity is presented in **Table 2**. Severity of each component varies depending on cause, extent of motor imbalance, and patient age.[23] Premature onset of disease distorts the entire hindfoot and forefoot anatomy because of pathologic growth of bones and makes a reconstructive procedure more demanding.[23]

Medial or plantarmedial peritalar subluxation describes the anatomic properties of a cavovarus foot. The posterior tibial tendon is strong and contracted, resulting in varus hindfoot alignment[24] and adduction of the midfoot and forefoot, whereas the peroneus brevis is weak or even absent. Because of varus malalignment at the heel, the pulling vector of the Achilles tendon becomes medialized, increasing the inversion moment and thus varus deformity.[25] In addition, a weak tibialis anterior muscle (eg, in Charcot-Marie-Tooth disease) becomes overpowered by the peroneus longus muscle, thus plantarflexing the first ray. The amount of plantarflexion at the first ray determines the height of the medial arch and thus the cavus component. Besides this mechanism, the plantarflexed first ray adds a rotatory malalignment of the forefoot, in other words, hyperpronation. The plantar fascia is generally contracted, adding to the adduction component and cavus deformity. Because there is a rotatory component in

Table 2
Causes of complex hindfoot varus deformity

Cause of Cavovarus	Pathology
Idiopathic	
Neurogenic	
- Cerebral disease	Cerebral palsy, stroke polio, tethered cord, amyotrophic
- Spinal cord disease	lateral sclerosis, Charcot-Marie-Tooth, spasticity of
- Peripheral neural disease	tibialis anterior or posterior, L5 motor radiculopahty
Residual clubfoot	
Traumatic	Lower leg compartment syndrome, talar neck malunion, peroneal nerve palsy, knee dislocations
Systemic inflammatory disease	Rheumatoid arthritis

cavovarus feet at the tarsus, the navicular moves into a more superior than medial position relative to the cuboid. The Chopart joint becomes torqued and fixes hindfoot varus. The evolution from supple to rigid cavovarus foot deformity is continuous. Once it has become rigid during stance phase, there is less shock absorption than, for example, in a valgus hindfoot deformity. The cavus deformity reduces the area of contact with the ground and increases localized pressure at the planta pedis, possibly leading to metatarsalgia and heel pain.[23] As a result of the previously mentioned biomechanical alterations, the lateral foot becomes overloaded,[26] and together with an impaired capacity of shock absorption due to subtalar locking and relative weakness of peroneus brevis, the risk of lateral ankle instability is increased. In addition, a fixed cavovarus deformity forces the talus into a varus tilt with chronic varus overload and possible evolution into medial ankle osteoarthritis.[2,12,16,27]

Normally forefoot-driven cavovarus deformity as explained previously is distinguished from hindfoot-driven variants. In the latter, the varus deformity represents the beginning of a pathologic process that contributes to further development of cavovarus deformity. Examples include lower leg compartment syndrome with deep posterior flexor contracture resulting in equinovarus and a malunited fracture of the talus.[5]

CLINICAL ASSESSMENT

The patient is examined barefoot both during walking and in a standing position. It is important to have the patient take off the trousers in order to estimate all lower limb axes. The alignments of both legs and hindfeet are evaluated. The goal of clinical evaluation is to assess the stability of the ankle joint and to obtain a detailed appreciation of the deformity type. Leg, hindfoot, midfoot, and forefoot deformities should be checked and assessed in order to estimate the rigidity and potential of possible correction. Throughout the clinical evaluation particular attention is paid to signs of concomitant pathologic conditions such as peroneal tendinopathy and lateral as well as medial instability, osteochondral lesions, osteoarthritis including ankle impingement, occult fractures, and neuropathy of the superficial peroneal nerve. However, in the following paragraphs the focus is on assessment of varus malalignment and ankle instability.

Inspection

Hindfoot alignment is observed during stance and includes inspection of soft-tissue conditions, for example, atrophy. Pelvic tilt, leg length discrepancies, and knee axis are

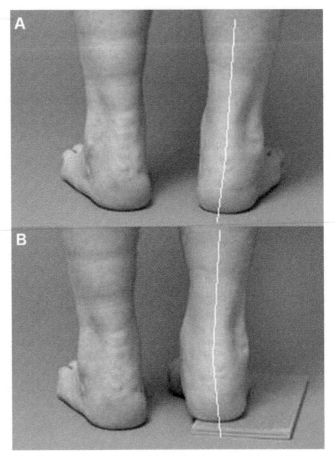

Fig. 1. The heels of a patient with a varus malalignment on the right side but physiologic hindfoot valgus of 0° to 5° on the left side (*A*). The Coleman block test reveals flexible hindfoot deformity (*B*).

assessed. Measurement of hindfoot alignment is performed while looking at the patient from behind (**Fig. 1**). The angle between long axis of the leg and axis of the calcaneus is measured. Normal values range from 0° neutral to 5° valgus. Any varus is pathologic.

The examiner could look for a peek-a-boo heel, as described by Manoli[28]: When examining the patient from the front, the visibility of the medial heel pad indicates the presence of hindfoot varus. The height of the medial longitudinal arch and the amount of first ray plantarflexion are noted, and special attention is paid to the position of the forefoot and midfoot under varus and valgus stress as well as pronation and supination. Analysis of gait and distribution of callosities at the plantar aspect may reveal dynamic components and could indicate regions that are overloaded.

Palpation

During palpation, special attention is paid to tender spots along the course of the medial and lateral ligament complexes around the ankle as well as along the joint lines of the ankle, subtalar, and Chopart joints. Tenderness along the peroneal tendons may indicate tendinopathy or partial rupture and needs specific imaging, for example, magnetic resonance imaging (MRI). Occasionally a prominent osteophyte formation points toward arthritic disorders. If local swelling is observed, palpation allows identification of joint effusion, tenosynovitis, or ganglion formation.

Function and Specific Tests

The flexibility of hindfoot varus—for example, in forefoot-driven hindfoot varus—can be tested by means of the Coleman block test (see **Fig. 1**).[29]

Range of motion (ROM) at the ankle, subtalar, and Chopart joints is assessed. Reduced ROM at any of those joints helps to identify the locus of rigidity and deformity. Reduced ROM at the ankle with concomitant equinus indicates a short gastrocnemius-soleus muscle complex. In order to assess the contribution of a short gastrocnemius-soleus complex, the so-called Silferskjöld test is performed (**Fig. 2**). It is important to rule out shortening of the Achilles tendon and contractures of the triceps surae because they may play an important role in correcting the hindfoot and

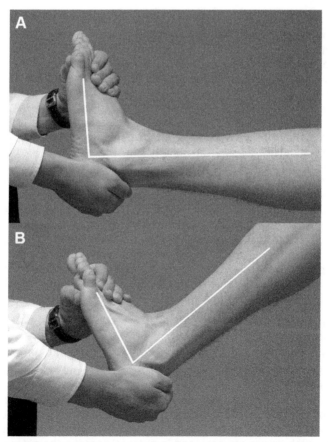

Fig. 2. The so-called Silferskjöld test to evaluate contracture of the gastrocnemius-soleus complex. With the knee held in maximum extension, dorsiflexion is minimal (A). When flexing the knee to 90° the dorsiflexion augments, indicating isolated contracture of the gastrocnemius muscle unit (B).

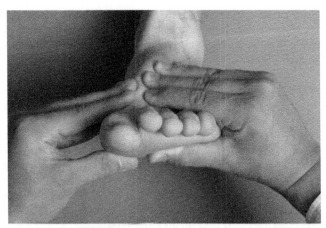

Fig. 3. Assessment of hyperpronation of the forefoot due to hyperactivity of the peroneus longus muscle.

in determining whether additional surgery should be performed. Hyperactivity of the peroneus longus, although debated, is tested as follows: The patient is examined in the sitting position and is asked to forcefully dorsiflex at the ankle joint with the knee in full extension. In this position the examiner places one thumb underneath the first metatarsal head and the other thumb underneath the second, third, and fourth metatarsal heads. The patient is then asked to maximally plantarflex the foot against resistance of the examiner. If pronation of the forefoot occurs with a strong plantarization of the first ray, hyperactivity of the peroneus longus muscle is present. Patients who plantarflex their foot without pronation of the forefoot are considered to have a normal activity of the peroneus longus muscle (**Fig. 3**).

Stability of the anterior talofibular and calcaneofibular ligaments is always compared with the contralateral side. The anterior drawer test (**Fig. 4**) is used to examine the anterior talofibular ligament, whereas the talar tilt (**Fig. 5**) assesses the stability of the calcaneofibular ligament. Valgus tilt allows evaluating integrity of the deltoid ligament. Any laxity or sign of generalized hypermobility should be evaluated.

Active muscle force against manual resistance allows documentation of each muscle group. Finally, the examination is completed with neurologic examination for sensation and reflexes. Bilateral absence of Achilles tendon reflexes may indicate the presence of peripheral neuropathy and requires additional neurologic workup.

RADIOGRAPHIC ASSESSMENT
Conventional Radiography

Standard anteroposterior and lateral views of the ankle under weight-bearing conditions are performed. In addition, the authors also recommend hindfoot alignment or long axial views to measure the amount of varus deformity. In order to rule out adjacent joint arthritis, dorsoplantar and lateral views of the foot are obtained. On the lateral view of the foot, the cavus deformity can be measured using various angles. Most commonly the talus–first metatarsal (Meary) and talocalcaneal angles as well as the calcaneal pitch angles are assessed in order to describe the deformity. On the mortise view, the congruency of the ankle joint can be judged and the lateral distal tibial angle (LDTA) measured (normal value 88°).[30] Varus tilt either due to medial tibial plafond erosion and arthritis or lateral ligament incompetence can easily be

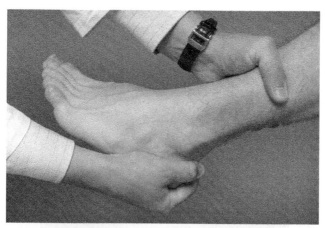

Fig. 4. Testing of the anterior talofibular ligament. The ankle is held in 20° plantarflexion and grasped with the dominant hand. With the nondominant hand, the tibia is fixed. Forced anterior translation is exerted with the dominant hand at the heel. Any increased anterior shift of the talus within the mortise when compared with the healthy side indicates ligament incompetence.

distinguished. Small but rounded ossicles found close to the fibular tip may indicate an old ligamentous avulsion injury.

Additionally, possible risk factors for chronic ankle instability, although more of academic interest, include an increased talar radius (normal: 18 mm), a small tibiotalar coverage (normal: 88°), and deeper frontal curvatures (normal: 1.0).[31–34]

Stress View

Stress views are rarely indicated but may be necessary in case of suspected instability but clinically not apparent laxity of the lateral ankle ligaments. Stress

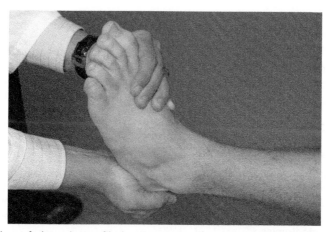

Fig. 5. Testing of the calcaneofibular ligament. The ankle is held in neutral or slight dorsiflexion and grasped with the dominant hand. With the nondominant hand, the tibia is fixed. Forced lateral tilt is exerted with the dominant hand at the heel. Any increased lateral opening of the talus within the mortise when compared with the healthy side indicates ligament incompetence.

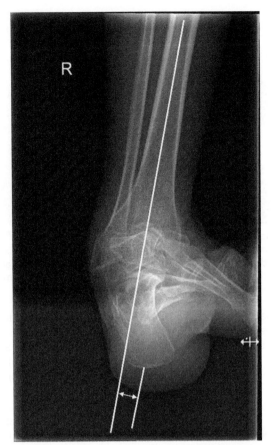

Fig. 6. Hindfoot view as described by Saltzman and el-Khoury.[40] The hindfoot is in significant varus deformity.

radiographs can be obtained manually or with the aid of a specific stress device. When performing the anterior drawer test, a subluxation of 9 mm or a difference greater than 5° to the healthy side indicates instability. When performing a talar tilt, a value of at least 10° or greater than 5° difference is suspicious for existing instability.[35–37] However, because of its moderate reliability, use of stress testing may be questionable.[38] The authors do not perform stress testing at their institution.

Hindfoot Assessment

Full-length anteroposterior and lateral views of the lower limb are used to identify the anatomic and mechanical axis of the knee, tibia, heel, and ankle. These views allow the measurement of the LDTA and TAS as well as the ability to find the center of rotation of angulation in case of tibial deformity, and they help in preoperative planning of osteotomies.[39]

Saltzman and el-Khoury[40] introduced the hindfoot view, a modification of the Cobey view (**Fig. 6**).[41,42] The superiority of the hindfoot view for visual judgment of the hindfoot alignment and its correlation to pedobarographic load distributions after total ankle replacement has been confirmed.[43] In addition, the hindfoot view has proven good-to-excellent intraobserver reliability. However, interobserver reliability is very low and is clearly surpassed when using a long axial view only.[44] One of the drawbacks of the hindfoot view is its susceptibility to rotatory malpositioning of the foot. Thus, the measurements obtained with the hindfoot view need to be interpreted with caution.[41] A far more reliable angle measurement can be done using the long axial view or the medial and lateral borders of the calcaneus.[45]

Whereas preoperative assessment of hindfoot alignment under weight-bearing conditions is done in a standardized fashion, there is not yet a technique available to do so under non–weight-bearing conditions, for example, during surgery. More recently, Min and Sanders[46] described varus-valgus referencing relative to the medial process of the posterior calcaneal tuberosity in the unloaded Mortise view. Its usefulness and feasibility will be the subject of future research.

Advanced Imaging

Nowadays, MRI and computed tomography (CT) allow precise three-dimensional depiction of the bones and soft tissues. Therefore, these technologies are mainly indicated for evaluation of the lateral ligamentous complex and concomitant pathologic conditions such as peroneal tendinopathy, osteochondral lesions, and/or osteoarthritis. MRI has been found to be highly specific in detecting lesions of the anterior talofibular (100%) and calcaneofibular (83%) ligaments; however, sensitivity is poor (56% and 50%, respectively).[47] Because of its superiority when compared with a simple arthro-CT, examination the authors perform CT only in selective cases, for example, to estimate the amount of fibular malrotation, to measure the true extent of osteochondral lesions of the talus, or to evaluate presence of a tarsal coalition.

CONSERVATIVE TREATMENT

Conservative treatment plays an important role when addressing chronic ankle instability. In the presence of postural abnormalities or mechanical deformities, for example in cavovarus foot, the value of a nonoperative treatment is questionable because it may not be effective enough in correcting rigid deformities and thus fail over time. However, some individuals will not allow themselves to be operated on, and for some, comorbidities increase health risks and outweigh the benefits of surgery. This group includes elderly patients and those with inadequately regulated diabetes mellitus, advanced peripheral vascular disease or cardiovascular disease, specific neurologic disorders, or respiratory disease.

Although conservative treatment does not address the underlying cause of a mechanically induced varus hindfoot deformity, it might be beneficial in cases of flexible varus deformity and when ligamentous insufficiency has been identified as the primary cause.

Conservative treatment should be followed for up to 6 months. If after a standardized nonoperative protocol there is no improvement, surgery may be considered.

Physical Therapy

Physical therapy has been shown to influence functional instability by improving proprioception, peroneal muscle preactivation, and eversion strength.[48–51] An aggressive stretching protocol is performed in order to lengthen the gastrocnemius-soleus unit and to reduce tension exerted through the Achilles tendon. By so doing, the inversion moment can be reduced and stability improved.

Braces

Braces can decrease severity and frequency of ankle sprains in athletes with chronic instability. Laced braces have been shown to be most effective.[52,53] In addition, improved stability can be achieved with taping. Although the inversion moments at the ankle are reduced by means of taping, the effect of taping is limited. It has been shown that almost 50% of the stabilizing effect is gone after 10 minutes of exercise.[54,55] However, proprioception might still remain improved due to other reflex mechanisms. Braces may also help to stretch the gastrocnemius-soleus unit.

Insoles and Orthoses

The primary goal of insoles and orthoses is to equalize pressure distribution and thus offload painful areas while supporting the medial arch. Lateral wedging may partially correct flexible hindfoot varus and decrease subjective instability.[26] Prefabricated products are available, but custom-made devices have advantages, especially in patients with rigid deformity. Additional support may be achieved with specific shoe modifications, for example increased width of the heel sole. In case of secondary degenerative changes, rocker-bottom soles could alleviate pain by reducing the propulsive work at the ankle joint.

APPROACHING THE PATIENT WITH VARUS ANKLE AND INSTABILITY

It is beyond the scope of this article to discuss in detail each surgical treatment of cavovarus deformity. The authors instead present conceptual thoughts in order to explain the approach to the patient with varus hindfoot deformity associated with chronic instability.

The goal of any reconstructive type of surgery is to achieve a plantigrade, fully functional, and stable foot. In order to choose the adequate treatment (eg, osteotomies, ligament reconstruction, fusions), surgeons should identify the apex and rigidity of deformity, assess associated muscle imbalances, and evaluate involvement and amount of joint degeneration.

Whenever possible, a joint-preserving approach should be considered.[56–61] The apex of deformity is found at the location where the malformation is most pronounced. Thus, for example, in the case of a hindfoot-driven cavovarus, the origin is found at the hindfoot with variable deformities found at the midfoot and forefoot.

The application of osteotomies, fusions, or a combination of both always depends on the severity of deformity. Normally, an oblique or Z-shaped calcaneal osteotomy is powerful enough to realign the heel in relation to the pulling vector of the Achilles tendon. In more severe varus deformity, realignment could be achieved by means of a laterally closing-wedge subtalar arthrodesis, and in extreme varus deformity subtalar fusion should even be combined with a lateral sliding calcaneal osteotomy.[62] In cavovarus feet, the anteromedial part of the ankle is overloaded because of deformity[16,24] and chronic lateral ankle instability.[12,13,63] A lateralizing calcaneal osteotomy unloads the medial ankle compartment[64] and might be considered in early stages of ankle osteoarthritis.[15] In contrast, subtalar arthrodesis exerts additional strain on the ankle joint, which already has or is at risk of degeneration.[56]

In a hindfoot-driven cavovarus deformity with subtle midfoot and forefoot malalignment, additional osteotomies at the forefoot may be preventable. However, in most cases an excessively plantarflexed and rigid first ray with consecutively increased medial arch and forefoot supination can be found. A majority of patients also demonstrate increased inclination of the first through fifth metatarsals with increased pressure underneath the corresponding metatarsal heads. Metatarsalgia is the result.

In such cases a dorsiflexion osteotomy of the first metatarsal, and sometimes first through third metatarsals, is performed.

Conversely, in forefoot-driven cavovarus, a dorsiflexion osteotomy of the metatarsals could be sufficient to correct the hindfoot varus moment as long as the tarsal deformity remains flexible.[65] The metatarsal osteotomy lowers the medial arch. If the longitudinal arch height cannot be lowered to the desired amount, an additional plantar fascia release should be considered.[66]

OSTEOTOMIES

The use of osteotomies in the treatment of ankle instability due to varus malalignment has recently gained new interest. The goal of osteotomies is to realign the hindfoot and to unload overstressed cartilaginous regions while adjusting the tension of the surrounding tendons and ligaments. Any type of osteotomy can be applied together with a combination of simple ligament repair or more sophisticated reconstructions.

As mentioned previously, when attempting to correct malalignment, the apex of deformity must be determined.[59]

In the absence of degenerative changes or in case of asymmetric osteoarthritis of the hindfoot, realignment surgery should be preferred over corrective arthrodesis in order to preserve joint motion at the hindfoot and to reduce abnormal stress transmissions through the midfoot and forefoot.[8,67,68]

Supramalleolar Osteotomy

A supramalleolar osteotomy is indicated in case of asymmetric ankle osteoarthritis or a malaligned distal tibial plafond. Depending on leg length, the osteotomy can be done either in a medial opening-wedge or lateral closing-wedge fashion. This procedure can be with or without a fibular osteotomy (**Fig. 7**).[8,27,68–76] However, in most cases the fibula is osteotomized as well. If the fibula is obviously overlong (eg, as seen after improper fracture fixation), the talar body cannot be brought into neutral position within the mortise. In such a situation the shortening of the fibula is a powerful means to realign the hindfoot. Fibular osteotomies can either be done in a Z-shaped or oblique fashion and should be fixed by means of a plate.

Although supramalleolar osteotomies have been described for the treatment of hemophilic ankles,[75] Takakura and colleagues[66,56] more recently introduced the concept of low tibial osteotomies in the treatment of primary osteoarthritis of the ankle. Eighteen patients with primary varus ankle osteoarthritis and medial joint narrowing but normal radiographic appearance of the lateral ankle compartment were included. Correction was achieved by means of a medial open-wedge osteotomy, which was filled with bone graft harvested either from the iliac crest or tibia. In all patients a fibular osteotomy was added. Just a few patients needed a repair of the lateral ligaments. All osteotomies united. Encouraged by the results obtained in this group, a few years later the same authors extended their indications to posttraumatic ankle arthritis.[67,68] However, in this series (including 9 patients with posttraumatic varus deformity), union was seen in all but 1 patient 2 months postoperatively.

Talar Osteotomies

In patients with clubfoot deformity, the talar head is positioned laterally to the midline axis but the forefoot is adducted and inclined with additional flexion at the talonavicular joint. A midfoot cavus is the result. In such patients, residual cavovarus deformity can be addressed by means of a lateral column shortening or by a talar neck osteotomy as proposed by Klaue.[77,78] The goal is to medialize the talar head and

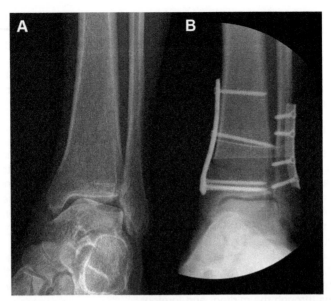

Fig. 7. A 50 year-old man had chronic lateral ankle instability and progressive pain due to medial ankle osteoarthritis. The preoperative anteroposterior view of the ankle (A) reveals a varus tilt of 15°. The lateral distal articular tibial angle measures 88° on the long leg views. The lateral half of the talar cartilage was intact and confirmed by arthroscopy. A medial open wedge osteotomy of the distal tibia corrected the lateral distal articular tibial angle to 92° in order to unload the medial compartment. In addition, an anatomic lateral ligament reconstruction with a gracilis tendon autograft, resection of osteophytes at the lateral gutter, and fibular shortening by 3 mm of the talus markedly realigned the ankle within the mortise (B).

move it inferior to correct both varus and cavus. The maximum shift achieved averages 10 mm. The osteotomy is done starting proximal lateral at the edge of the cartilage and driven medially. If not enough lengthening is obtained, a bone graft can be interposed. One of the most dangerous risks is avascular necrosis of the talar head. This risk might explain why this osteotomy has not become popular among orthopaedic surgeons. Klaue proposed a lateral Ollier approach to preserve blood supply to the talar head. In severe deformity, a lateralizing calcaneal osteotomy may be necessary. Early results of the talar osteotomy showed satisfactory results.

Despite such congenital pathologic conditions as clubfoot deformity, posttraumatic malunions of the talar neck after fracture are observed in up to 32% of cases. Most of these pertain to unrecognized injuries, secondary dislocation after nonoperative treatment of displaced fractures, and inadequate surgical reduction or fixation.[79] The malunion forces the talar head medially and cranially in relation to the neck, causing anterior ankle impingement, varus deformity of the neck, and hindfoot malalignment, as well as restricted subtalar joint motion. The results after osteotomy in cases of preserved cartilage are acceptable.[80,81]

Calcaneal Osteotomies

Valgus calcaneal osteotomy in lateral instability should be performed for dynamic hindfoot varus to correct abnormal inversion stress through the medialized force of the Achilles tendon, which acts in this configuration as an inverter.[4] One of the goals is to change the tendon pull direction to bring it to more of a pronator function. The other effect is that the foot is corrected during heel strike.[5]

Calcaneal osteotomies are well-known in orthopaedic surgery and have become widely used. This procedure is a powerful tool to correct rigid but not forefoot-driven hindfoot varus. However, by lateralizing the heel, the medial column could become stressed and painful. In such a situation an elevating (dorsiflexing) first metatarsal osteotomy should be considered.[29,82] If hindfoot malalignment is driven by a flexible or fixed forefoot deformity, therapy must always include correction of the pathologic condition in the forefoot.

A calcaneal osteotomy can be done in various ways. Dwyer[83,84] popularized a curved shaped and lateral closing-wedge osteotomy. The problem with this osteotomy is that it allows only small corrections and through calcaneal shortening the lever and moment arm for the Achilles tendon become shorter and weaker, respectively.[24,64]

A more powerful form of correction is the lateral sliding osteotomy (**Fig. 8**). The transverse osteotomy is performed perpendicular to the long axis of the calcaneus from posterosuperior to anteroinferior. The tuberosity can be displaced laterally by 10 mm. Two 6.5-mm displacements are used to fix the osteotomy and provide rotatory stability. In cavovarus deformity, a slight cranial displacement of 10 mm allows reduction of the cavus component. Good to excellent results were reported in cavovarus feet when a lateral sliding osteotomy was combined with a first metatarsal osteotomy.[61]

The most powerful osteotomy by far is the Z-shaped osteotomy of the calcaneus.[82] This procedure allows a correction in three planes. Because of its scarf-like design, it offers intrinsic stability while the tuber is shifted laterally. Lengthening of the calcaneus, shortening, internal or external rotation, and inversion and eversion can be added by means of resecting or adding bone blocks into the osteotomy site. It has been shown that in cavovarus feet, a Z-shaped osteotomy restores force distribution across the varus ankle while reducing peak pressures. Because of lateralization of the ground contact point, the pressure within the tibiotalar joint shifts laterally. In the presence of normal subtalar joint mobility, with calcaneal osteotomies, peak pressures alterations in the tibiotalar joint are improved.

The authors use a simple lateral sliding or Z-shaped lateral sliding osteotomy and may add a lateral ligament reconstruction to correct varus and to restore stability. When considering a lateral ligament repair,[85] the osteotomy is performed first. A lateral curved incision is done. Subcutaneous dissection is performed carefully in order to avoid the sural nerve. Periosteal stripping is kept minimal. The cranial and plantar borders of the tuber calcanei are identified, followed by insertion of blunt Hohmann retractors. Afterward, the cut is performed by means of an oscillating saw. The nondominant hand is placed on the medial aspect of the posterior part of the calcaneus. This maneuver allows immediate control of the penetrating saw blade. At times, periosteal incision on the medial, dorsal, and plantar osteotomy site must be done with a scalpel to allow lateral shifting of the bone. The osteotomy is fixed using two 6.5-mm partially threaded cancellous screws. Usually sufficient lateralization is achieved without the need of wedging. Lateral closing-wedge osteotomy is reserved for additional curved calcaneal deformities.

In case of slight degeneration of the ankle joint associated with chronic lateral ligament instability, Lee and colleagues[15] recommend a release of the deltoid ligament, augmentation of the lateral ligaments[86] combined with a lateralizing osteotomy of the calcaneus. The goal is to even stress loading at the talar cartilage and, of course, to delay progression of osteoarthritis. In the series by Lee and colleagues,[15] good stability was found in 9 of the 11 patients. Treatment failed for 2

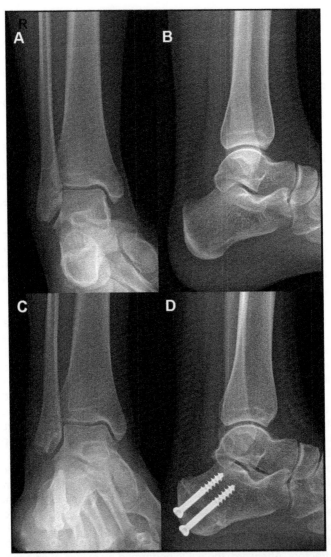

Fig. 8. Conventional radiographs (preoperative, *A, B*; postoperative, *C, D*) of a 15-year-old girl with recurrent lateral ankle sprains. A modified Broström procedure together with a lateralizing calcaneal osteotomy was performed. One year postoperatively, the patient was able to completely resume sports activities.

patients. Both showed a pronounced preoperative talar tilt of 11° and 12°, respectively. Overall results were promising at a mean follow-up time of 22 months.

Midfoot and Forefoot Osteotomies

Excessive pronation in the forefoot drives the hindfoot into supination.[8,9,69] A flexible plantarflexed first ray may arise from hyperactivity of the peroneus longus, which can be decreased by means of a peroneus longus to brevis transfer.[8,9]

Otherwise fixed plantarflexion of the metatarsals, for example as seen in idiopathic cavovarus foot, can be addressed by a dorsiflexion osteotomy. Dorsiflexion osteotomies may involve a single metatarsal or more metatarsals. Larger plantarflexion deformities might be better addressed using a fusion of the first tarsometatarsal joint.[5]

In forefoot-driven hindfoot varus, the deformity is caused by a rigid and massively plantarflexed first ray. In such a situation a dorsiflexion osteotomy of the proximal first metatarsal bone is recommended.[29,87,88] Vienne and colleagues[9] published the results of a consecutive series of patients with cavovarus deformity and recurrent ankle instability. All patients revealed a failed prior ligament stabilization surgery. The plantarflexed first ray and hindfoot varus were flexible. Each patient was clinically detected to have a hyperactivity of the peroneus longus muscle. All were successfully treated by means of a lateralizing calcaneal osteotomy and peroneus longus to brevis transfer. In half of the patients, a Broström procedure[85,89–93] was added to address lateral ligament insufficiency. All patients showed good results with subjective and objective lateral stability.

ADVANCED OSTEOARTHRITIS AT THE HINDFOOT AND STRATEGIES

In contrast to deformities that allow preservation of the joints, more severe and rigid deformity or end-stage osteoarthritis may be better addressed by arthrodesis. In the case of an intact and well-aligned ankle joint but arthritic and deformed subtalar and Chopart joint, a corrective triple arthrodesis could be considered. The authors use a modified and calcaneocuboidal joint–sparing triple arthrodesis technique (**Fig. 9**).[94] Besides an increased risk of ankle degeneration,[56] one must be aware of the risk of nonunion, which has been reported to range between 2% and 33%. The highest risk has been found in patients with neuromuscular disease. In contrast, once fusion is complete and solid and the foot plantigrade, outcomes are satisfying.[95–98]

Advanced stages of ankle osteoarthritis lead to less favorable outcomes, even after adequate foot and ankle realignment and lateral ligament reconstruction.[99] In such cases performance of an ankle arthrodesis or implantation of a total joint replacement are to be anticipated.

DYNAMIC BALANCING—TRANSFERS AND LENGTHENING

Peroneal muscle imbalance with impaired inversion strength is likely to be present in cavovarus feet. The peroneus brevis muscle is weak, whereas the peroneus longus may reveal hyperactivity. A pronatory moment is exerted at the forefoot because of increased plantarflexion of the first ray. The compensatory hindfoot varus cannot be halted by the action of peroneus brevis muscle. In this situation the most important lateral and dynamic stabilizer, the peroneus brevis, should be reinforced and the pathologic action of the peroneus longus abolished. The transfer of the peroneus longus to brevis tendon adds dynamic support to the lateral ankle. A lateral transfer of the tibialis anterior tendon to either the lateral cuneiform or cuboid is advocated in severe cases, provided the tibialis anterior muscle has sufficient strength (M4–M5 required).[100]

Equinus deformity may contribute to lateral ankle instability because the congruency of the ankle is minimal in plantarflexion. In this situation, stability of the joint depends on integrity of lateral ligaments, and muscle balance only enhances the susceptibility to varus thrusts. Ankle dorsiflexion may be sufficiently improved after correction of the talo–first metatarsal angle; however, if dorsiflexion does not exceed 5°, subsequent Achilles tendon lengthening or release of the gastrocnemius should be considered.

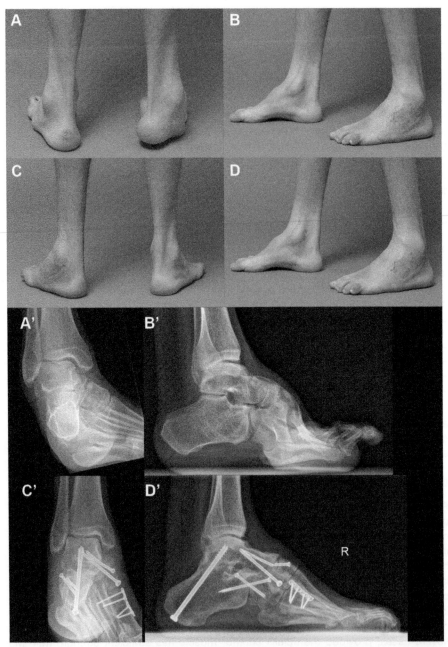

Fig. 9. An 18-year-old man had severe bilateral and rigid cavovarus feet suffered from associated chronic lateral ankle instability. Note the remarkable varus and cavus foot deformity (preoperative clinical photographs (*A, B*) and X-rays (*A', B'*). Surgical correction was performed by means of a Steindler release, posterior tibial tendon- and Achilles tendon lengthening, a dorsal closing wedge osteotomy of the first metatarsal, and triple arthrodesis. Intraoperatively, no remaining instability was found. Thus, a lateral ligament reconstruction was not necessary. One year postoperatively ([*C, D*] clinical photographs; [*C', D'*] X-rays), a plantigrade foot is present. The patient continues with sports without concerns about pain and with full stability.

LATERAL LIGAMENT REPAIR OR RECONSTRUCTION

The scientific literature confirms the effectiveness of lateral ankle repair or reconstruction for the treatment of chronic ankle instability. The primary aim of surgical therapy is to restore the integrity of ligaments. However, application of surgical therapy in patients with unstable varus ankle, especially cavovarus foot, remains unclear. Sammarco and Taylor[61] treated patients who had cavovarus foot pathology without adding a lateral ankle ligament reconstruction and reported good to excellent clinical results. Vienne and colleagues[9] reported on patients with cavovarus foot deformity who had had chronic ankle instability after previously failed surgeries. The varus malalignment was corrected by a calcaneal osteotomy, and dynamic balancing was achieved using a peroneus longus to brevis transfer. In half of the patients, an additional lateral ankle ligament reconstruction was performed because of persisting instability. At an average follow-up of 37 months, all patients were satisfied and American Orthopaedic Foot and Ankle Society (AOFAS) hindfoot scores improved from 57 to 87 points.[9] Conversely, Fortin and colleagues[16] reported complete resolution of pain and improved stability in all patients who were treated by lateral ankle ligament reconstruction combined with realignment surgery.

Whereas functional instability in the absence of static hindfoot malalignment can successfully be addressed by means of nonoperative measures,[101,102] obvious deformities need surgical correction. Symptoms are relieved by hindfoot realignment in case of varus deformity without the need of additional ligament repair. In a retrospective series by Sammarco and Taylor[60] of 21 ankles in 15 patients with cavovarus foot, 5 available for follow-up presented with instability as the primary concern. All were treated with combined hindfoot and forefoot osteotomy for the correction of deformity. Outcome assessed by AOFAS score was excellent in all patients except one in which follow-up was complicated by deep venous thrombosis and delayed union of the fourth metatarsal osteotomy.[60] The number of patients, however, does not allow concrete conclusions as to whether ligament repair should be added or not.

Based on these facts and in contrast to simple chronic ankle instability without varus deformity, the answer regarding whether ligament reconstruction in patients with cavovarus is necessary has not yet been found.

Ligament Repair and Augmentation

The ideal patient with regard to an anatomic and direct ligament repair with or without local augmentation has mild to moderate lateral ankle instability without deformity and reveals viable ligament tissue quality, absence of hyperlaxity, and a normal body mass index.

The technique of anatomic ligament repair was first introduced by Broström in 1966[89] and was subsequently modified by others. Karlsson and colleagues[103] described advancement of the ligament into the fibula whereas Gould and colleagues[86] and Kuner and colleagues[104] described a ligamentous augmentation by means of the extensor retinaculum or fibular periosteal sleeve, respectively.

Anatomic repair demonstrates durable, good to excellent results in 80% to 90% of patients after 26 years.[86,105–108] Nonetheless, the results in continuing or recurrent instability are less favorable.[103,106,109] Larger size and body weight, hyperlaxity, and increased physical demands during work and/or in sports impair outcome.[103,106,109,110] Inadequate reconstruction of the anterior talofibular ligament leads to elongation and insufficiency and increases the stress on the cervical and interosseus ligament as well. Because of incompetence of the anterior talofibular ligament, the cervical ligament could tear and lead to subtalar instability. Inadequate reconstruction of the calcaneofibular ligament results in persisting pain and increased varus thrust at the ankle joint.[111]

Ligament Reconstructions Using Grafts

In obese individuals and in patients with hyperlaxity or prior failed lateral stabilization, more limiting and nonanatomic types of reconstructions can be considered. However, these indications are rare. The concept is based on a complete or partial tenodesis of the peroneus brevis tendon after rerouting.[112–115] Although good and excellent outcomes after nonanatomic repairs have been reported, there are some serious drawbacks, for example, restricted subtalar motion, residual ankle instability, and increased risk of secondary osteoarthritis, making the routine use of such reconstruction questionable.[10,116–118] Another drawback of nonanatomic reconstruction is the higher rate of complications due to a more extensile soft-tissue dissection. Delayed wound healing has been found in 4% of patients as opposed to 1.6% in patients who have been treated by an anatomic repair. Nerve injuries have also been found more frequently in patients after nonanatomic reconstruction versus anatomic reconstruction (nonanatomic reconstruction, 10%; anatomic repair, 4%; anatomic reconstruction, 2%).[119] In order to reduce the risks, more recently, percutaneous techniques were introduced.[120,121]

Current anatomic reconstruction of lateral ankle ligaments use either hamstring or plantaris tendon grafts, which are rerouted in order to replace the anterior talofibular and calcaneofibular ligaments.[117,122–127]

The results of open and anatomic ligament reconstructions using grafts are promising. Coughlin and colleagues[127] in a series of 28 patients described subjective satisfaction as excellent in 86% and good in the remaining 14%, with an improvement in mean AOFAS score from 57 points preoperatively to 98 points after a follow-up of 2 years. Subtalar motion was not or minimally reduced as shown earlier in anatomic reconstructions by Paterson and colleagues,[125] Coughlin and colleagues,[127] and Hintermann and Renggli,[124] who used semitendinosus or gracilis grafts. It seems that anatomic reconstructions could lead to better long-term outcomes and reduced rates of subtalar degeneration. Even patients with hyperlaxity do well and reveal good outcomes. This result is interesting because it does away with the former belief that only nonanatomic reconstructions could achieve adequate stability in patients with hyperlaxity.[127] One patient had irritation of the sural nerve, and only 2 showed superficial cellulitis that resolved after oral administration of antibiotics. The series did not include patients who required hindfoot varus correction. Hintermann and Renggli[124] reported similar results in a series of 52 patients who had had an anatomic transfer of the plantaris tendon. Two of these patients required additional calcaneal osteotomy for hindfoot varus. After an average follow-up of 3.5 years, AOFAS score of 98 points was reached with 98% of patients reporting a good to excellent outcome.[124] Direct comparison between anatomic and nonanatomic ligament reconstructions is difficult because of different scoring systems and techniques used. However, Krips and colleagues[128–130] showed an advantage of anatomic repair in the long-term follow-up with higher scores and improved function and stability as well as decreased rates of revision and osteoarthritis. To the authors' knowledge there is no single prospective and randomized study that investigates nonanatomic versus anatomic reconstructions.

The authors prefer an open or percutaneous anatomic technique using a gracilis autograft. The technique has recently been described in detail by Klammer and colleagues.[121]

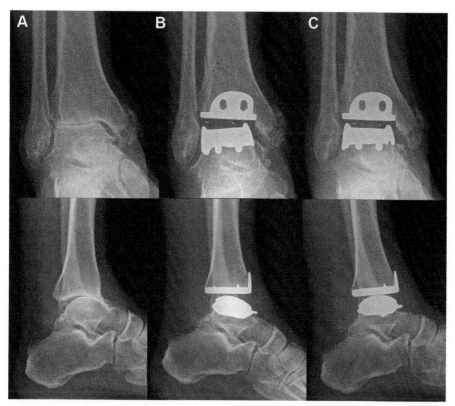

Fig. 10. A 50-year-old patient had had a total ankle replacement because of primary ankle osteoarthritis. Preoperative radiographs show advanced joint degeneration with anterior subluxation of the talus but no varus tilting (*A*). The postoperative radiography after a few days after implantation of the prosthesis shows talar tilting due to acute postoperative lateral ligament insufficiency (*B*). Balancing was restored with anatomic lateral ligament reconstruction using a gracilis autograft and increased inlay thickness (*C*).

TOTAL ANKLE REPLACEMENT IN THE UNSTABLE VARUS ANKLE

The success of total ankle replacement depends not only on design but also on anatomic hindfoot alignment and proper ligament balancing (**Fig. 10**). Edge loading of the polyethylene is a risk factor for early failure.[131–134] Therefore, a physiologic hindfoot position of 0° to 5° valgus should be attempted in all cases. Whereas Wood and Deakin[135] described an increased failure rate in ankles with a preoperative malalignment of more than 15° varus, Hobson and colleagues[134] reported safe and reliable results in patients who had a well-aligned total ankle replacement but who had had a preoperative varus ankle deformity up to 30°. Similar results were obtained by Kim and colleagues[136] in patients with a preoperative varus between 10° and 22°.

In contrast, Coetzee[137] recommended ankle fusion in patients with varus deformities greater than 20° because of the high failure rate of total ankle replacement in this patient category.

In case of a varus deformity located at the tibial plafond but congruent ankle configuration (talar tilt <10°), the joint line should be reoriented by performing a tibial bone cut that runs perpendicular to the mechanical axis of the tibia and parallel to the floor. This step might be followed by a medial release of the deltoid or distal translation of the medial malleolus.[136,138] If the height of the tibial cut exceeds the maximum thickness of the inlay, in other words if the varus deformity of the tibial plafond is greater than (5° to) 10°, an additional supramalleolar osteotomy is required.[71,72] This situation corresponds to stage 1 varus ankle according to Frank Alvine's classification. In stage 1, varus is induced by medial tibial erosion but absence of relevant ligament instability.[139]

In case of an anatomically oriented tibial plafond but incongruent talus within the mortise (talus tilts within mortise), the latter must first be restored. According to the Alvine classification, progression into stage 2 is characterized by lateral ligament insufficiency and medial and lateral ectopic bone formation that may inhibit anatomic placement of the talus within the mortise. The medial and lateral gutters are liberated from osteophytes in order to allow realignment of the talus. Medial tightness may inhibit reduction.[139] Thus, ligament balancing is done by releasing the deltoid ligament or by performance of a medial malleolar lengthening osteotomy.[138,139] Persisting lateral ankle joint gaping of more than 5° requires an additional anatomic lateral ligament reconstruction as previously described.[137] Alternatively, when ligament insufficiency is caused by an overlong fibula or in the presence of subfibular impingement, a fibular shortening osteotomy could be considered.[136]

In a well-aligned total ankle replacement with full restoration of joint congruence but persisting hindfoot varus, further extraarticular correction is needed.[136,138] This correction may be achieved with a lateral sliding calcaneal osteotomy or with subtalar or triple arthrodesis, depending on joint degeneration or in case of Alvine stage 3 varus ankle (medial malleolar bone erosion combined with a subluxation of the subtalar joint).[138,139]

SUMMARY

Varus ankle associated with instability can be simple or complex. Multiple underlying diseases may contribute to this complex pathologic entity. These conditions should be recognized when attempting proper decision-making. Treatment options range from conservative measures to surgical reconstruction. Whereas conservative treatment might be a possible approach for patients with simple varus ankle instability, more complex instabilities require extensive surgical reconstructions. However, adequate diagnostic workup and accurate analysis of varus ankle instability provide a base for the successful treatment outcome.

REFERENCES

1. Larsen E. Static or dynamic repair of chronic lateral ankle instability. A prospective randomized study. Clin Orthop 1990;(257):184–92.
2. Scranton PE Jr, McDermott JE, Rogers JV. The relationship between chronic ankle instability and variations in mortise anatomy and impingement spurs. Foot Ankle Int 2000;21(8):657–64.
3. Van Bergeyk AB, Younger A, Carson B. CT analysis of hindfoot alignment in chronic lateral ankle instability. Foot Ankle Int 2002;23(1):37–42.
4. Strauss JE, Forsberg JA, Lippert FG 3rd. Chronic lateral ankle instability and associated conditions: a rationale for treatment. Foot Ankle Int 2007;28(10):1041–4.
5. Younger AS, Hansen ST Jr. Adult cavovarus foot. J Am Acad Orthop Surg 2005; 13(5):302–15.
6. Tarr RR, Resnick CT, Wagner KS, et al. Changes in tibiotalar joint contact areas following experimentally induced tibial angular deformities. Clin Orthop Relat Res 1985;(199):72–80.

7. Ting AJ, Tarr RR, Sarmiento A, et al. The role of subtalar motion and ankle contact pressure changes from angular deformities of the tibia. Foot Ankle 1987;7(5):290–9.
8. Pagenstert GI, Hintermann B, Barg A, et al. Realignment surgery as alternative treatment of varus and valgus ankle osteoarthritis. Clin Orthop Relat Res 2007;462: 156–68.
9. Vienne P, Schoniger R, Helmy N, et al. Hindfoot instability in cavovarus deformity: static and dynamic balancing. Foot Ankle Int 2007;28(1):96–102.
10. Colville MR. Surgical treatment of the unstable ankle. J Am Acad Orthop Surg 1998;6(6):368–77.
11. Valderrabano V, Horisberger M, Russell I, et al. Etiology of ankle osteoarthritis. Clin Orthop Relat Res 2009;467(7):1800–6.
12. Harrington KD. Degenerative arthritis of the ankle secondary to long-standing lateral ligament instability. J Bone Joint Surg Am 1979;61(3):354–61.
13. Valderrabano V, Hintermann B, Horisberger M, et al. Ligamentous posttraumatic ankle osteoarthritis. Am J Sports Med 2006;34(4):612–20.
14. Sugimoto K, Samoto N, Takakura Y, et al. Varus tilt of the tibial plafond as a factor in chronic ligament instability of the ankle. Foot Ankle Int 1997;18(7):402–5.
15. Lee HS, Wapner KL, Park SS, et al. Ligament reconstruction and calcaneal osteotomy for osteoarthritis of the ankle. Foot Ankle Int 2009;30(6):475–80.
16. Fortin PT, Guettler J, Manoli A 2nd. Idiopathic cavovarus and lateral ankle instability: recognition and treatment implications relating to ankle arthritis. Foot Ankle Int 2002;23(11):1031–7.
17. Biedert R. Anterior ankle pain in sports medicine: aetiology and indications for arthroscopy. Arch Orthop Trauma Surg 1991;110(6):293–7.
18. Frahm R, Fritz H, Drescher E. [Pathologic changes in the hindfoot angle following fracture of the calcaneus]. Rofo 1989;151(2):192–5 [in German].
19. Varner KE, Michelson JD. Tarsal coalition in adults. Foot Ankle Int 2000;21(8): 669–72.
20. Barg A, Elsner A, Hefti D, et al. Total ankle arthroplasty in patients with hereditary hemochromatosis. Clin Orthop Relat Res 2011;469:1427–35.
21. Hintermann B, Nigg BM. [Movement transfer between foot and calf in vitro]. Sportverletz Sportschaden 1994;8(2):60–6 [in German].
22. Ledoux WR, Shofer JB, Ahroni JH, et al. Biomechanical differences among pes cavus, neutrally aligned, and pes planus feet in subjects with diabetes. Foot Ankle Int 2003;24(11):845–50.
23. Aminian A, Sangeorzan BJ. The anatomy of cavus foot deformity. Foot Ankle Clin 2008;13(2):191–8,v.
24. Krause F, Windolf M, Schwieger K, et al. Ankle joint pressure in pes cavovarus. J Bone Joint Surg Br 2007;89(12):1660–5.
25. Grumbine NA, Santoro JP. The tendo Achillis as it relates to rearfoot position. A new classification for evaluation of calcaneal stance position. Clin Podiatr Med Surg 1990;7(2):203–16.
26. Manoli A 2nd, Graham B. The subtle cavus foot, "the underpronator". Foot Ankle Int 2005;26(3):256–63.
27. Harstall R, Lehmann O, Krause F, et al. Supramalleolar lateral closing wedge osteotomy for the treatment of varus ankle arthrosis. Foot Ankle Int 2007;28(5): 542–8.
28. Manoli A 2nd, Smith DG, Hansen ST Jr. Scarred muscle excision for the treatment of established ischemic contracture of the lower extremity. Clin Orthop 1993;292:309–14.

29. Coleman SS, Chesnut WJ. A simple test for hindfoot flexibility in the cavovarus foot. Clin Orthop Relat Res 1977;(123):60–2.
30. Paley D. Correction of limb deformities in the 21st century. J Pediatr Orthop 2000;20(3):279–81.
31. Frigg A, Frigg R, Hintermann B, et al. The biomechanical influence of tibio-talar containment on stability of the ankle joint. Knee Surg Sports Traumatol Arthrosc 2007;15(11):1355–62.
32. Frigg A, Magerkurth O, Valderrabano V, et al. The effect of osseous ankle configuration on chronic ankle instability. Br J Sports Med 2007;41(7):420–4.
33. Frigg A, Nigg B, Hinz L, et al. Clinical relevance of hindfoot alignment view in total ankle replacement. Foot Ankle Int 2010;31(10):871–9.
34. Magerkurth O, Frigg A, Hintermann B, et al. Frontal and lateral characteristics of the osseous configuration in chronic ankle instability. Br J Sports Med 2010; 44(8):568–72.
35. Beynnon BD, Webb G, Huber BM, et al. Radiographic measurement of anterior talar translation in the ankle: determination of the most reliable method. Clin Biomech (Bristol, Avon) 2005;20(3):301–6.
36. Garber MB. Diagnostic imaging and differential diagnosis in 2 case reports. J Orthop Sports Phys Ther 2005;35(11):745–54.
37. Harper MC. Stress radiographs in the diagnosis of lateral instability of the ankle and hindfoot. Foot Ankle 1992;13(8):435–8.
38. Frost SC, Amendola A. Is stress radiography necessary in the diagnosis of acute or chronic ankle instability? Clin J Sport Med 1999;9(1):40–5.
39. Knupp M, Pagenstert G, Valderrabano V, et al. [Osteotomies in varus malalignment of the ankle]. Oper Orthop Traumatol 2008;20(3):262–73 [in German].
40. Saltzman CL, el-Khoury GY. The hindfoot alignment view. Foot Ankle Int 1995;16(9): 572–6.
41. Johnson JE, Lamdan R, Granberry WF, et al. Hindfoot coronal alignment: a modified radiographic method. Foot Ankle Int 1999;20(12):818–25.
42. Cobey JC. Posterior roentgenogram of the foot. Clin Orthop Relat Res 1976;(118): 202–7.
43. Frigg A, Nigg B, Davis E, et al. Does alignment in the hindfoot radiograph influence dynamic foot-floor pressures in ankle and tibiotalocalcaneal fusion? Clin Orthop Relat Res 2010;468(12):3362–70.
44. Reilingh ML, Beimers L, Tuijthof GJ, et al. Measuring hindfoot alignment radiographically: the long axial view is more reliable than the hindfoot alignment view. Skeletal Radiol 2010;39(11):1103–8.
45. Buck FM, Hoffmann A, Mamisch-Saupe N, et al. Hindfoot alignment measurements: rotation-stability of measurement techniques on hindfoot alignment view and long axial view radiographs. AJR Am J Roentgenol 2011;197(3):578–82.
46. Min W, Sanders S. The use of the mortise view of the ankle to determine hindfoot alignment: technique tip. Foot Ankle Int 2010;31(9):823–7.
47. Chandnani VP, Harper MT, Ficke JR, et al. Chronic ankle instability: evaluation with MR arthrography, MR imaging, and stress radiography. Radiology 1994;192(1): 189–94.
48. Freeman MA, Dean MR, Hanham IW. The etiology and prevention of functional instability of the foot. J Bone Joint Surg Br 1965;47(4):678–85.
49. Freeman MA. Instability of the foot after injuries to the lateral ligament of the ankle. J Bone Joint Surg Br 1965;47(4):669–77.
50. Lofvenberg R, Karrholm J, Sundelin G, et al. Prolonged reaction time in patients with chronic lateral instability of the ankle. Am J Sports Med 1995;23(4):414–7.

51. Wilkerson GB, Pinerola JJ, Caturano RW. Invertor vs. evertor peak torque and power deficiencies associated with lateral ankle ligament injury. J Orthop Sports Phys Ther 1997;26(2):78–86.
52. Gross MT, Liu HY. The role of ankle bracing for prevention of ankle sprain injuries. J Orthop Sports Phys Ther 2003;33(10):572–7.
53. Verhagen AP, de Bie RA, Lenssen AF, et al. Impact of quality items on study outcome. Treatments in acute lateral ankle sprains. Int J Technol Assess Health Care 2000;16(4):1136–46.
54. Laughman RK, Carr TA, Chao EY, et al. Three-dimensional kinematics of the taped ankle before and after exercise. Am J Sports Med 1980;8(6):425–31.
55. Robbins S, Waked E, Rappel R. Ankle taping improves proprioception before and after exercise in young men. Br J Sports Med 1995;29(4):242–7.
56. Wetmore RS, Drennan JC. Long-term results of triple arthrodesis in Charcot-Marie-Tooth disease. J Bone Joint Surg Am 1989;71(3):417–22.
57. Gould N. Surgery in advanced Charcot-Marie-Tooth disease. Foot Ankle 1984;4(5):267–73.
58. Ward CM, Dolan LA, Bennett DL, et al. Long-term results of reconstruction for treatment of a flexible cavovarus foot in Charcot-Marie-Tooth disease. J Bone Joint Surg Am 2008;90(12):2631–42.
59. LaClair SM. Reconstruction of the varus ankle from soft-tissue procedures with osteotomy through arthrodesis. Foot Ankle Clin 2007;12(1):153–76, x.
60. Sammarco GJ, Taylor R. Combined calcaneal and metatarsal osteotomies for the treatment of cavus foot. Foot Ankle Clin 2001;6(3):533–43, vii.
61. Sammarco GJ, Taylor R. Cavovarus foot treated with combined calcaneus and metatarsal osteotomies. Foot Ankle Int 2001;22(1):19–30.
62. Haddad SL, Myerson MS, Pell RF 4th, et al. Clinical and radiographic outcome of revision surgery for failed triple arthrodesis. Foot Ankle Int 1997;18(8):489–99.
63. Rieck B, Reiser M, Bernett P. [Post-traumatic arthrosis of the upper ankle joint in chronic insufficiency of the fibular ligament]. Orthopade 1986;15(6):466–71 [in German].
64. Krause FG, Sutter D, Waehnert D, et al. Ankle joint pressure changes in a pes cavovarus model after lateralizing calcaneal osteotomies. Foot Ankle Int 2010;31(9):741–6.
65. Leeuwesteijn AE, de Visser E, Louwerens JW. Flexible cavovarus feet in Charcot-Marie-Tooth disease treated with first ray proximal dorsiflexion osteotomy combined with soft tissue surgery: a short-term to mid-term outcome study. Foot Ankle Surg 2010;16(3):142–7.
66. Bacardi BE, Alm WA. Modification of the Gould operation for cavovarus reconstruction of the foot. J Foot Surg 1986;25(3):181–7.
67. Takakura Y, Takaoka T, Tanaka Y, et al. Results of opening-wedge osteotomy for the treatment of a post-traumatic varus deformity of the ankle. J Bone Joint Surg Am 1998;80(2):213–8.
68. Takakura Y, Tanaka Y, Kumai T, et al. Low tibial osteotomy for osteoarthritis of the ankle. Results of a new operation in 18 patients. J Bone Joint Surg Br 1995;77(1):50–4.
69. Pagenstert G, Knupp M, Valderrabano V, et al. Realignment surgery for valgus ankle osteoarthritis. Oper Orthop Traumatol 2009;21(1):77–87.
70. Roukis TS. Corrective ankle osteotomies. Clin Podiatr Med Surg 2004;21(3):353–70, vi.

71. Stamatis ED, Cooper PS, Myerson MS. Supramalleolar osteotomy for the treatment of distal tibial angular deformities and arthritis of the ankle joint. Foot Ankle Int 2003;24(10):754–64.
72. Stamatis ED, Myerson MS. Supramalleolar osteotomy: indications and technique. Foot Ankle Clin 2003;8(2):317–33.
73. Mangone PG. Distal tibial osteotomies for the treatment of foot and ankle disorders. Foot Ankle Clin 2001;6(3):583–97.
74. Cheng YM, Chang JK, Hsu CY, et al. Lower tibial osteotomy for osteoarthritis of the ankle. Gaoxiong Yi Xue Ke Xue Za Zhi 1994;10(8):430–7.
75. Pearce MS, Smith MA, Savidge GF. Supramalleolar tibial osteotomy for haemophilic arthropathy of the ankle. J Bone Joint Surg Br 1994;76(6):947–50.
76. Graehl PM, Hersh MR, Heckman JD. Supramalleolar osteotomy for the treatment of symptomatic tibial malunion. J Orthop Trauma 1987;1(4):281–92.
77. Klaue K. Planovalgus and cavovarus deformity of the hind foot. A functional approach to management. J Bone Joint Surg Br 1997;79(6):892–5.
78. Klaue K. Hindfoot issues in the treatment of the cavovarus foot. Foot Ankle Clin 2008;13(2):221–7, vi.
79. Rammelt S, Zwipp H. Talar neck and body fractures. Injury 2009;40(2):120–35.
80. Monroe MT, Manoli A 2nd. Osteotomy for malunion of a talar neck fracture: a case report. Foot Ankle Int 1999;20(3):192–5.
81. Rammelt S, Winkler J, Heineck J, et al. Anatomical reconstruction of malunited talus fractures: a prospective study of 10 patients followed for 4 years. Acta Orthop 2005;76(4):588–96.
82. Malerba F, De Marchi F. Calcaneal osteotomies. Foot Ankle Clin 2005;10(3):523–40, vii.
83. Dwyer FC. The present status of the problem of pes cavus. Clin Orthop Relat Res 1975;(106):254–75.
84. Dwyer FC. Osteotomy of the calcaneum for pes cavus. J Bone Joint Surg Br 1959;41-B(1):80–6.
85. Paden MH, Stone PA, McGarry JJ. Modified Brostrom lateral ankle stabilization utilizing an implantable anchoring system. J Foot Ankle Surg 1994;33(6):617–22.
86. Gould N, Seligson D, Gassman J. Early and late repair of lateral ligament of the ankle. Foot Ankle 1980;1(2):84–9.
87. Paulos L, Coleman SS, Samuelson KM. Pes cavovarus. Review of a surgical approach using selective soft-tissue procedures. J Bone Joint Surg Am 1980;62(6):942–53.
88. Chilvers M, Manoli A 2nd. The subtle cavus foot and association with ankle instability and lateral foot overload. Foot Ankle Clin 2008;13(2):315–24, vii.
89. Broström L. Sprained ankles. VI. Surgical treatment of "chronic" ligament ruptures. Acta Chir Scand 1966;132(5):551–65.
90. Broström L. Sprained ankles. 3. Clinical observations in recent ligament ruptures. Acta Chir Scand 1965;130(6):560–9.
91. Broström L. [Ankle sprains]. Lakartidningen 1967;64(16):1629–44 [in Swedish].
92. Broström L. Sprained ankles. V. Treatment and prognosis in recent ligament ruptures. Acta Chir Scand 1966;132(5):537–50.
93. Broström L, Sundelin P. Sprained ankles. IV. Histologic changes in recent and "chronic" ligament ruptures. Acta Chir Scand 1966;132(3):248–53.
94. Sammarco VJ, Magur EG, Sammarco GJ, et al. Arthrodesis of the subtalar and talonavicular joints for correction of symptomatic hindfoot malalignment. Foot Ankle Int 2006;27(9):661–6.

95. Mann DC, Hsu JD. Triple arthrodesis in the treatment of fixed cavovarus deformity in adolescent patients with Charcot-Marie-Tooth disease. Foot Ankle 1992;13(1):1–6.
96. Saltzman CL, Salamon ML, Blanchard GM, et al. Epidemiology of ankle arthritis: report of a consecutive series of 639 patients from a tertiary orthopaedic center. Iowa Orthop J 2005;25:44–6.
97. Sangeorzan BJ, Smith D, Veith R, et al. Triple arthrodesis using internal fixation in treatment of adult foot disorders. Clin Orthop Relat Res 1993;(294):299–307.
98. Wukich DK, Bowen JR. A long-term study of triple arthrodesis for correction of pes cavovarus in Charcot-Marie-Tooth disease. J Pediatr Orthop 1989;9(4):433–7.
99. Irwin TA, Anderson RB, Davis WH, et al. Effect of ankle arthritis on clinical outcome of lateral ankle ligament reconstruction in cavovarus feet. Foot Ankle Int 2010;31(11):941–8.
100. Medical Research Council. Aids to the examination of the peripheral nervous system. Memorandum No. 45. London, England: HMSO; 1976:1.
101. DiGiovanni CW, Brodsky A. Current concepts: lateral ankle instability. Foot Ankle Int 2006;27(10):854–66.
102. Freedman LS, Jenkins AI, Jenkins DH. Carbon fibre reinforcement for chronic lateral ankle instability. Injury 1988;19(1):25–7.
103. Karlsson J, Bergsten T, Lansinger O, et al. Reconstruction of the lateral ligaments of the ankle for chronic lateral instability. J Bone Joint Surg Am 1988;70(4):581–8.
104. Kuner EH, Goetz K. [Surgical therapy of chronic instability of the upper ankle joint using periostal bridle-plasty]. Orthopade 1986;15(6):454–60 [in German].
105. Karlsson J, Bergsten T, Lansinger O, et al. Surgical treatment of chronic lateral instability of the ankle joint. A new procedure. Am J Sports Med 1989;17(2):268–73 [discussion: 273–4].
106. Karlsson J, Bergsten T, Lansinger O, et al. Lateral instability of the ankle treated by the Evans procedure. A long-term clinical and radiological follow-up. J Bone Joint Surg Br 1988;70(3):476–80.
107. Rudert M, Wulker N, Wirth CJ. Reconstruction of the lateral ligaments of the ankle using a regional periosteal flap. J Bone Joint Surg Br 1997;79(3):446–51.
108. Bell SJ, Mologne TS, Sitler DF, et al. Twenty-six-year results After Broström procedure for chronic lateral ankle instability. Am J Sports Med 2006;34:976–8.
109. Karlsson J, Eriksson BI, Bergsten T, et al. Comparison of two anatomic reconstructions for chronic lateral instability of the ankle joint. Am J Sports Med 1997;25(1):48–53.
110. Girard P, Anderson RB, Davis WH, et al. Clinical evaluation of the modified Brostrom-Evans procedure to restore ankle stability. Foot Ankle Int 1999;20(4):246–52.
111. Coughlin MJ, Schenck RC Jr, Grebing BR, et al. Comprehensive reconstruction of the lateral ankle for chronic instability using a free gracilis graft. Foot Ankle Int 2004;25(4):231–41.
112. Watson-Jones R. Recurrent forward dislocation of the ankle joint. J Bone Joint Surg Br 1952;134:519.
113. Evans DL. Recurrent instability of the ankle; a method of surgical treatment. Proc R Soc Med 1953;46(5):343–4.
114. Chrisman OD, Snook GA. Reconstruction of lateral ligament tears of the ankle. An experimental study and clinical evaluation of seven patients treated by a new modification of the Elmslie procedure. J Bone Joint Surg Am 1969;51(5):904–12.
115. Elmslie R. Recurrent subluxation of the ankle joint. Proc R Soc Med 1934;37:364–7.
116. Bahr R, Pena F, Shine J, et al. Biomechanics of ankle ligament reconstruction. An in vitro comparison of the Broström repair, Watson-Jones reconstruction, and a new anatomic reconstruction technique. Am J Sports Med 1997;25(4):424–32.
117. Colville MR, Marder RA, Zarins B. Reconstruction of the lateral ankle ligaments. A biomechanical analysis. Am J Sports Med 1992;20(5):594–600.

118. Rosenbaum D, Becker HP, Wilke HJ, et al. Tenodeses destroy the kinematic coupling of the ankle joint complex. A three-dimensional in vitro analysis of joint movement. J Bone Joint Surg Br 1998;80(1):162–8.

119. Sammarco VJ. Complications of lateral ankle ligament reconstruction. Clin Orthop Relat Res 2001;(391):123–32.

120. Maquieira GJ, Moor BK, Espinosa N. Technique tip: percutaneous Chrisman-Snook lateral ankle ligament reconstruction. Foot Ankle Int 2009;30(3):268–70.

121. Klammer G, Schlewitz G, Stauffer C, et al. Percutaneous lateral ankle stabilization: an anatomical investigation. Foot Ankle Int 2011;32(1):66–70.

122. Colville MR, Grondel RJ. Anatomic reconstruction of the lateral ankle ligaments using a split peroneus brevis tendon graft. Am J Sports Med 1995;23(2):210–3.

123. Colville MR. Reconstruction of the lateral ankle ligaments. Instr Course Lect 1995; 44:341–8.

124. Hintermann B, Renggli P. [Anatomic reconstruction of the lateral ligaments of the ankle using a plantaris tendon graft in the treatment of chronic ankle joint instability]. Orthopade 1999;28(9):778–84 [in German].

125. Paterson R, Cohen B, Taylor D, et al. Reconstruction of the lateral ligaments of the ankle using semi-tendinosis graft. Foot Ankle Int 2000;21(5):413–9.

126. Anderson ME. Reconstruction of the lateral ligaments of the ankle using the plantaris tendon. J Bone Joint Surg Am 1985;67(6):930–4.

127. Coughlin MJ, Matt V, Schenck RC Jr. Augmented lateral ankle reconstruction using a free gracilis graft. Orthopedics 2002;25(1):31–5.

128. Krips R, Brandsson S, Swensson C, et al. Anatomical reconstruction and Evans tenodesis of the lateral ligaments of the ankle. Clinical and radiological findings after follow-up for 15 to 30 years. J Bone Joint Surg Br 2002;84(2):232–6.

129. Krips R, van Dijk CN, Halasi PT, et al. Long-term outcome of anatomical reconstruction versus tenodesis for the treatment of chronic anterolateral instability of the ankle joint: a multicenter study. Foot Ankle Int 2001;22(5):415–21.

130. Krips R, van Dijk CN, Halasi T, et al. Anatomical reconstruction versus tenodesis for the treatment of chronic anterolateral instability of the ankle joint: a 2- to 10-year follow-up, multicenter study. Knee Surg Sports Traumatol Arthrosc 2000;8(3):173–9.

131. Espinosa N, Walti M, Favre P, et al. Misalignment of total ankle components can induce high joint contact pressures. J Bone Joint Surg Am; 92(5):1179–87.

132. Haskell A, Mann RA. Ankle arthroplasty with preoperative coronal plane deformity: short-term results. Clin Orthop Relat Res 2004;(424):98–103.

133. Wood PL, Prem H, Sutton C. Total ankle replacement: medium-term results in 200 Scandinavian total ankle replacements. J Bone Joint Surg Br 2008;90(5):605–9.

134. Hobson SA, Karantana A, Dhar S. Total ankle replacement in patients with significant pre-operative deformity of the hindfoot. J Bone Joint Surg Br 2009;91(4):481–6.

135. Wood PL, Deakin S. Total ankle replacement. The results in 200 ankles. J Bone Joint Surg Br 2003;85(3):334–41.

136. Kim BS, Choi WJ, Kim YS, et al. Total ankle replacement in moderate to severe varus deformity of the ankle. J Bone Joint Surg Br 2009;91(9):1183–90.

137. Coetzee JC. Surgical strategies: lateral ligament reconstruction as part of the management of varus ankle deformity with ankle replacement. Foot Ankle Int 2010;31(3):267–74.

138. Kim BS, Knupp M, Zwicky L, et al. Total ankle replacement in association with hindfoot fusion: outcome and complications. J Bone Joint Surg Br 2010;92(11):1540–7.

139. Coetzee JC. Management of varus or valgus ankle deformity with ankle replacement. Foot Ankle Clin 2008;13(3):509–20, x.

Distal Tibial Varus

Douglas Beaman, MD*, Richard Gellman, MD

KEYWORDS
- Complex deformity • Distal tibial varus deformity
- Distraction osteogenesis • Gradual correction
- Limb shortening

The focus of this article is the correction of distal tibial varus deformities utilizing gradual techniques and distraction osteogenesis. Distraction osteogenesis is the formation of new bone after an osteotomy is completed using tension-lengthening techniques.

Distraction osteogenesis employed with multiplanar ring external fixation is a minimally invasive method that is advantageous when there is a compromised soft tissue envelope or compromised bone. Current ring fixation techniques allow gradual simultaneous multiplanar correction that can be difficult to obtain with acute correction.

Gradual correction of deformity allows for postoperative assessment to confirm that correction has been obtained, and adjustments can be made as needed to optimize an accurate final correction; acute corrections are determined intraoperatively. Gradual correction with distraction osteogenesis also offers the ability to regain limb length. Gradual correction minimizes acute stretch injuries to neurovascular structures and the soft tissue envelope. This is particularly important in the varus to valgus correction.

In our clinical experience, distraction osteogenesis is typically chosen over acute correction when the deformity is complex, involving an oblique plane, multiplane, or rotational component. In addition, gradual correction is chosen when an isolated varus deformity is moderate to severe, generally greater than 15°, and the ability to confidently correct the deformity acutely is compromised. Prior infection or soft tissue envelope compromise are also relative indications that favor distraction osteogenesis with percutaneous techniques, avoiding greater surgical dissection and the use of internal fixation devices.

Associated ankle arthritis and ligamentous instability are other considerations, because the ankle joint can be distracted and stabilized in conjunction with distal tibial boney deformity correction. The use of ring fixation may allow for the patient to be more functional during the healing period; a ring fixator allows at least partial weight bearing during recovery. This enables patients to more safely transfer and

The authors have nothing to disclose.
Summit Orthopedic, 501 North Graham Street, Suite 250, Portland, OR 97227-1651, USA
* Corresponding author.
E-mail address: dnbeaman@gmail.com

Foot Ankle Clin N Am 17 (2012) 83–93
doi:10.1016/j.fcl.2011.11.002
1083-7515/12/$ – see front matter © 2012 Elsevier Inc. All rights reserved.

foot.theclinics.com

eliminates the potential for loss of correction or collapse if patients are noncompliant with weight-bearing instructions.

Distraction osteogenesis is preferred when acute correction would likely result in significant shortening or would create an unstable osteotomy. The ultimate decision to utilize distraction osteogenesis techniques includes a careful evaluation of the patient and the patient's ability to care for a ring fixator. Because patient involvement is required during treatment, we favor an organized team approach in which all involved are familiar with the ring fixation techniques, including the orthopedic surgeon, office staff, physical therapist, orthotist, and hospital staff.

NATURAL HISTORY

The consequences of tibial malalignment remain controversial. There is not a clear understanding of the degree or type of deformity that creates a symptomatic patient. Based on clinical and basic science studies, there are multiple factors involved in creating patients' symptoms in the face of tibial deformity.

The primary clinical problem with malalignment is asymmetric loading of joints, with the ankle joint the primary concern in distal tibia varus. Secondary arthritic change may occur. Lateral foot pain may develop secondary to lateral column overload, compensatory subtalar valgus, and subtalar arthrosis.

Clinical studies evaluating the natural history of tibial malunion have been performed in long-term follow-up of tibia fractures; however, most studies include a limited number of patients. There is a lack of consensus on the degree of angulation and its effect on knee and ankle function. There may be bias given the potential that patients lost to follow-up had undergone realignment surgery owing to symptomatic malunion.[1–7]

Puno and colleagues[8] evaluated 28 tibia fractures with 8 years of follow-up. Varus ankle malalignment greater than 4° correlated with a poor ankle score. The overall joint orientation was more important than fracture angulation alone. Twenty-nine percent of the ankles developed significant joint space narrowing in their study and 50% of ankles were symptomatic, whereas only 19% of knees were symptomatic, and 68% of ankles had decreased range of motion, varying from mild to near-absent motion.

Milner and colleagues[6] confirmed that arthritic changes developed in 58% of patients who healed in greater than 5° of angular deformity compared to 31% with less than 5°. They also found an increase of osteoarthritis of the subtalar joint.

Because most distal tibial malunions are posttraumatic deformities, it is essential to evaluate ankle and subtalar joint arthrosis from the inciting trauma that is distinct from altered joint loading and progressive joint wear owing to the malunion. Direct joint arthrosis can occur from an ankle or pilon fracture, dislocations or sprains, or prolonged immobilization in casts. Depending on the extent of arthritis, the surgeon should caution patients that despite a successful deformity correction, improvement in pain relief and function may be limited.

In addition to the coronal plane deformity found in distal tibia varus, patients may also have significant translational, rotational, or sagittal plane deformity. Translation may accentuate or diminish the effects of the angulation, depending on its direction. Significant rotational deformity may be highly symptomatic depending on the patient's activity level and ability to accept a foot progression angle different than the uninjured side.

Sagittal plane deformity has important effects on ankle joint motion and stability. A procurvatum deformity limits ankle dorsiflexion and interferes with even simple activities of daily living, such as walking and stair climbing, whereas recurvatum causes the talus and foot to sublux anteriorly.

Ting and colleagues,[9] in a cadaveric study, demonstrated that distal third tibial deformities create greater decreases in ankle contact area than proximal and mid shaft tibial deformities. This was particularly noted in the procurvatum deformities.

Subtalar joint motion compensates for distal tibia varus by eversion in the hindfoot. As subtalar joint motion becomes restricted, there is a decrease in the ankle contact area with all tibial deformities. This is more pronounced in the varus tibia than the valgus tibia because the subtalar joint normally has less eversion than inversion. Varus of the distal tibia also moves ground contact forces medially, which again limits eversion of the subtalar joint.

PUBLISHED RESULTS OF DEFORMITY CORRECTION

The majority of published data on distal tibial deformity correction involves acute correction with internal fixation techniques employing a variety of osteotomy techniques. Most have small numbers and variable follow-up, but offer some important clinical observations on the degree of correction that can be achieved acutely, the presence of osteoarthritis in the ankle, subtalar joint arthrosis, and ligamentous laxity of the ankle. Several of the authors recommend slight, approximately 2° to 5°, of overcorrection.

Graehl and colleagues[10] evaluated patients with distal tibial varus malunions. They recommended the dome osteotomy for coronal plane malunion correction. In our experience, the dome osteotomy has provided either an anteroposterior (AP) or sagittal plane angulation correction up to 10°. However, more severe deformity correction can be technically difficult.

Pearce and associates[11] reported on osteotomy for hemophilic arthropathy of the ankle with valgus deformity. Procedures were performed without fibular osteotomy. The patients experienced significant pain relief and a decrease in frequency and severity of intra-articular hemorrhage. The use of a fibular osteotomy for a varus correction is typically required to achieve correction of the tibial deformity; however, consideration can be given for tibial osteotomy alone if the tibial deformity is a result of a tibial malunion without fibular deformity and correction can be achieved without requiring significant translation.

Cheng and co-workers[12] reported on osteotomies with moderate ankle arthritis; they were able to achieve significant improvement. All patients showed medial joint space widening postoperatively with a gradual increase and improvement in arthrosis. Stamatis and colleagues[13] performed osteotomies in patients with ankle arthritis. Postoperatively, there was no evidence of arthritic progression at 3 years and patients experienced significant pain relief. Tanaka and associates[14] reported on varus ankles with osteoarthritis corrected with opening wedge osteotomy. The more severely arthritic joints and patient's with a preoperative varus tilt of the talus greater than 10° demonstrated less improvement. Pagenstert and co-workers[15] reported on 35 patients with complex deformities. Ninety-one percent of the patients had additional procedures based on deformity. The overall success rate was satisfactory. Fibular osteotomy was considered based on the malleolar angle or rotational deformity or syndesmotic subluxation.

The varus tilt of the distal tibia seems to be a likely factor in the development of chronic lateral ankle instability and the development of ankle arthritis. Indeed, Sugimoto and colleagues[16] reported that the varus tilt of the tibial plafond is more prevalent in patients with chronic lateral ankle ligament instability than in patients with acute ligament sprains. Lee and associates[17] demonstrated that patients with varus ankles often have valgus heel alignment, and this may have an important role if varus deformity correction is performed in the face of a fixed valgus heel. A valgus postoperative heel alignment was associated with postoperative subfibular pain. In this study, a higher degree of talar tilt—greater than 10°—was associated with a less satisfactory postoperative result. Also recommended was consideration for a gradual correction in patients with a valgus heel alignment and a varus distal tibia to avoid the potential for creating a significant hindfoot valgus deformity after supramalleolar correction.

SURGICAL PLANNING

The surgical plan for correction of a distal tibia varus deformity requires an understanding of normal limb alignment, a method to accurately measure the deformity, and assessment of possible compensatory foot deformities. Once the surgeon understands the tibial deformity, he or she must decide the optimal location of the osteotomy, what type to perform, whether to include the fibula, and whether to correct acutely or gradually. This article briefly describes normal alignment, deformity analysis, osteotomy planning and gradual correction with the Taylor spatial frame. More extensive references are listed.[15,18–20]

Normal Alignment

In the frontal or coronal plane, normal alignment of the lower extremity is defined as the mechanical axis, a straight line that extends from the center of the hip through the center of the knee, to the center of the ankle joint. The mechanical axis inferior to the ankle extends down through the center of the talus and ends approximately 1 cm medial to the center vertical axis of the calcaneal tuberosity.

On a standing AP radiograph of the tibia, the lateral distal tibial angle (LDTA) is the frontal plane joint angle measured in degrees that is used to determine whether the articular surface of the distal tibia is in varus, normal, or valgus alignment. The LDTA is measured at the intersection of anatomic axis of the tibia and a line parallel to the distal tibial plafond on the lateral side. The anatomic axis is determined by taking 2 midpoints in the diaphysis of a long bone and connecting them with a straight line. The mechanical axis and the anatomic axis of the tibia are exactly parallel, however, the anatomic axis is, on average, 4 mm medial to the mechanical axis.

The normal average LDTA is 89° (normal range, 86°–92°). Conceptually, therefore, the goal of surgical treatment for a distal tibia varus deformity is to make the distal tibia articular surface perpendicular and centered just medial to the tibial anatomic axis. To measure alignment distal to the ankle, the hindfoot alignment view radiograph is used.[21] It is a weight-bearing radiograph that allows observation of the distal tibia, ankle joint, and calcaneal tuberosity on a single view. This radiograph requires a specialized mounting box to angle the radiographic plate 20° from the vertical plane. The long axial view is another radiograph that is non–weight bearing that visualizes the tibia, subtalar joint, and calcaneal tuberosity, and does not require a special mounting box.

It is important to understand that malalignment in distal tibial varus deformities can occur from malunion in the distal tibia bone, intra-articular wear in the ankle joint, or from ligamentous laxity creating talar tilt. The visualization of intra-articular wear and ligamentous laxity are best seen on weight-bearing radiographs and, thus, should be obtained whenever feasible.

The normal distal tibial angle in the sagittal plane is 80° measured anteriorly and thus termed the anterior distal tibia angle. The mid tibial line intersects the midpoint of the talar dome and the lateral talar process, although the exact location varies with the position of ankle dorsiflexion or plantarflexion.

Tibial external or internal rotation is measured clinically using the foot–thigh angle. A perpendicular line extending from the tibial tubercle normally matches the axis of the second toe. Rotation is usually matched to the contralateral asymptomatic side. If there is significant deformity in the foot, rotation can be determined by palpation of the medial and lateral malleolus at the ankle instead. Complex rotational deformities may require bilateral axial computed tomography scans of the proximal and distal tibias for more accurate measurement.

Standing, full-length, lower extremity AP and lateral radiographs from the hip to the ankle are obtained if there is deformity above the distal tibial region or a limb length discrepancy. The weight-bearing AP foot radiograph is measured for talo–first metatarsal angle, navicular coverage, and joint subluxation or arthritis. The lateral foot view is measured for talo–first metatarsal angle, calcaneal pitch, and joint subluxation or arthritis. Comparison weight-bearing radiographs of the contralateral, asymptomatic limb should be obtained for preoperative planning.

Deformity Measurement

In common orthopedic nomenclature, the point where the proximal and distal anatomic or mechanical axes intersect is termed the apex of the deformity. Because the distal tibia is too short to form an anatomic axis, a line is drawn from the center of the distal tibial surface, using the previously described LDTA measured from the contralateral limb or the normal average of 89°. This intersects with the anatomic axis of the tibia shaft to give the degree and location of the varus deformity.

The apex is the optimal location for the osteotomy and axis to correct the deformity, so it also has been termed the center of rotation of angulation (CORA). If the CORA does not seem to fall at the apex, then there has likely been shortening and/or translation as the malunion formed. The same method is then used to determine any sagittal plane malunion on the lateral radiograph using the contralateral anterior distal tibial angle or 80° normal average.

Distal tibial varus deformities that have the CORA at or near the joint are described as juxta-articular. These are common after distal tibial growth arrest or collapse after ankle pilon fractures. The osteotomy must be made proximal to the CORA to avoid the ankle joint. In this case, angulation correction alone results in a lateral translational deformity. Therefore, the distal tibial segment must be translated medially to correctly realign the limb axis.

Correction with the osteotomy at the CORA avoids secondary translations. However, it is often impossible to perform an osteotomy at the CORA for distal tibial varus and the operative plan must include medial translation necessary to achieve an adequate correction. This is an important principle and one usually ignored when varus deformities are acutely corrected with opening or closing wedge osteotomies and plate fixation.

COMPENSATORY DEFORMITIES

Compensatory deformities are common in the foot. Varus deformities of the distal tibia usually are compensated in the subtalar joint and the forefoot. The subtalar joint compensates for a distal tibia varus deformity by moving into an everted position. Because the average eversion in the subtalar joint is 10°, varus deformities of greater than 10° cause symptoms from weight bearing on the lateral border of the foot.

In the forefoot, tibial varus deformity is compensated by forefoot pronation. This is seen as a valgus forefoot or a plantarflexed first ray when the patient's foot is examined in the non–weight-bearing position. The need to correct the compensatory deformities depends on their extent and the degree of arthrosis. The goal after correction of the distal tibial varus is to leave a plantigrade foot. If the subtalar joint and medial column remain flexible, then hindfoot and first ray fusions or osteotomies are not necessary.

Certain cases of muscle imbalance may cause the hindfoot to be in varus below a distal tibia varus deformity owing to weakness or absence of peroneal muscle strength. The forefoot is usually affected as well, and remains in a supinated position. The muscle imbalance needs to be addressed with release or tendon transfer, possibly in a staged fashion to avoid wound complications. Rigid hindfoot deformity without significant joint arthrosis should be corrected with either medial displacement calcaneal osteotomy for heel valgus or lateral displacement, Dwyer-type valgus producing osteotomy for heel varus. Avoiding subtalar fusion is preferable because it increases the risk of arthritic change in the ankle.

Forefoot valgus is corrected with first metatarsal dorsiflexion osteotomy, and possible plantar fascia release. Forefoot varus may require first tarsometatarsal arthrodesis or correction through the talonavicular and calcaneal–cuboid joints if there is a more severe, rigid deformity. When performing gradual deformity correction of the distal tibia, immediate correction of the foot deformity is usually completed before application of the external fixator.

Osteotomy Location

Once the CORA is defined, the location of osteotomy then becomes more straight-forward. There must be adequate distance between the osteotomy and the ankle joint to allow placement of smooth wires if gradual correction with Ilizarov techniques are chosen or for placement of screw fixation if acute correction with plate and screws is utilized. Other considerations are regions of poor bone at the CORA that may prohibit the surgeon from placing his osteotomy, where delayed healing could be a significant risk. Similarly, placing an osteotomy in a region of significant soft tissue trauma, such as bone covered only by a healed, split-thickness skin graft may cause the surgeon to change the location of the osteotomy owing to concerns of poor bone healing or wound dehiscence and infection.

Decision Making: Immediate or Gradual Correction?

Immediate correction of deformity is indicated for mild deformities without major shortening, soft tissue loss, or neurovascular compromise. Mild is defined as a 5° to 10° uniplanar deformity in healthy appearing bone. A dome osteotomy may be performed with a combination of internal and external fixation. Gradual correction is preferred for deformities greater than 10° or multiplanar deformities. Malunions associated with significant shortening also require gradual correction to restore leg length. Poor soft tissue and neurovascular risks and compensatory foot deformities, along with patient-related factors, including the inability to maintain minimal weight bearing, are additional indications for gradual correction with the Ilizarov technique, because multiplanar external fixation is strong enough to allow ambulation and transfers.

Osteotomy Types and Techniques

The optimal osteotomy technique preserves periosteal blood supply and minimizes thermal bone necrosis. Ilizarov's principles emphasize the preservation of intramedullary blood supply, but more recent studies with the multiple drill hole or Gigli saw techniques have shown no major difference in osteotomy healing rates whether intramedullary blood supply is preserved or disrupted. Corticotomy or multiple drill hole osteotomy yields more blood vessels bridging the distraction gap than an osteotomy done with an oscillating saw.[20] The preferred osteotomy technique varies with the anatomic location. A multiple drill hole technique is preferred in the diaphyseal region of the distal third of the tibia, whereas a Gigli saw osteotomy is preferred in the more distal metadiaphyseal and supramalleolar areas.

For drill hole osteotomy, a 1-cm, vertical skin incision is made just medial to the tibialis anterior tendon. The drill hole should be made about 5 mm medial to the most anterior point on the anterior tibial cortical ridge. This avoids heat necrosis to the thick, dense, anterior cortical bone. Through the single anterior starting drill hole, multiple drill holes through the posterior tibial cortex are created working from medial to lateral with a 3.8- or 4.8-mm drill bit. Copious saline irrigation is applied to the drill bit and firm, controlled drill pressure is applied to maximize cutting efficiency and minimize heating of the bone. The osteotomy is completed with a 1-cm, sharp osteotome directed along the posterior, medial, and lateral cortices; careful elevation of the medial and lateral periosteum is performed so that it is not injured by the osteotome.

A Gigli saw osteotomy requires 2 or 3 incisions, depending on the level of osteotomy. For tibial metadiaphyseal osteotomies that do not include the fibula, 2 horizontal incisions are utilized. One is made posteromedial and one anterior. Careful elevation of the periosteum is made on all 3 surfaces of the tibia before passing a heaving suture between the 2 incisions from the posterior incision around the posterior tibia and then up to the anterior incision along the lateral face of the tibia. The suture pass requires 2 long, narrow clamps. A curved or right angle clamp delivers the suture end around the posterior tibia cortex. The Gigli saw is pulled through by the suture, taking care to protect the periosteum, tendons, and neuro-vascular structures. Firm, long strokes are applied to the handles of the Gigli saw to prevent binding in the bone and this aspect of the procedure requires careful attention. Once the saw has reached the medial tibial face, the retractors are adjusted to protect the medial periosteum, the medial tibia cortex cut is completed, and the saw can be cut with a pin cutter for easy removal.

For osteotomies in the metaphysis, where both the distal tibia and fibula are cut, 3 incisions are required, 1 posteromedial, 1 anteromedial, and 1 directly lateral over the fibula. Elevation of the periosteum occurs along the surfaces of both the tibia and fibula anterior and posterior and the saw is passed from medial to lateral, beginning the osteotomy through the fibula first. Because the level of this osteotomy is so close to the joint, we often place a temporary smooth wire through the tibia and fibula at the level of the planned osteotomy to serve as a guide for the Gigli saw blade. This prevents the osteotomy from accidentally heading toward the articular surface of the ankle joint where there still needs to be sufficient space for wire fixation in the distal tibia.

The focal dome osteotomy is useful for immediately correcting distal tibial deformity when the CORA is at or just proximal to the ankle joint. The osteotomy is made as distal as possible, allowing for fixation, to take advantage of metaphyseal bone healing. For frontal plane deformities, a 6-mm half pin is placed in the distal tibia below the level of the osteotomy (at the CORA). Several 4.8-mm drill holes are made through a curved radiolucent jig or through connecting cubes (Rancho Cube, Smith & Nephew, Memphis, TN, USA) to form the dome shape, and the bone between the drilled holes is cut with a sharp osteotome. An acute correction is performed and the osteotomy may be translated by rotation of the osteotome within the osteotomy. As detailed, translation is necessary to realign the mechanical axis because the osteotomy is not made through the CORA. The osteotomy is stabilized with 1 or 2 screws.

The half pin can be left in place for stabilization of the distal tibial ring if combined with Ilizarov external fixation.

Fibular Osteotomy

Fibular osteotomy is indicated for fibular deformity associated with a tibial deformity. When the fibular deformity is similar to the tibial deformity (level and extent), the fibular and tibial osteotomies are made at the same level. An oblique fibular osteotomy is made with a small sagittal saw or the multiple drill hole technique. If the fibula is not deformed and there is an isolated tibial deformity (eg, after pilon fracture with fibula fixed and tibial malunion), the tibia may be osteotomized without a fibular osteotomy. Fibular osteotomy distal to the tibial osteotomy is indicated when translation is required for realignment.

Taylor Spatial Frame

The Taylor Spatial Frame is useful for gradual correction of distal tibial deformities because of the precision afforded with the Internet-based program. This system enables simultaneous 6-axis deformity correction using the 6-strut platform. Traditional Ilizarov techniques require accurate placement of a hinge at the CORA along the axis of the varus deformity. Frame modifications are then required to correct other aspects of the deformity. These frame modifications become prohibitively time consuming, especially when correcting rotation or translation deformity compared with use of the Taylor spatial software. The Taylor spatial frame is also significantly stronger than the Ilizarov frame, which decreases the chance of frame hardware failure during correction in heavier patients.

Frame application

A tibial base frame is applied proximal to the deformity by assembling 2 Taylor spatial rings with 120- or 150-mm threaded rods and securing it to the tibia shaft with a single transverse smooth 1.8-mm Ilizarov wire and two 6-mm hydroxyapatite coated half pins off each ring. Multiplanar fixation placement is followed to maximize strength. Next, a Taylor spatial ring is mounted exactly parallel to the distal tibia just above the ankle joint to allow clear radiographic visualization of the joint. This is often technically demanding and patience should be exercised to get this ring perfectly aligned. Fixation is usually achieved with 3 to 4 smooth or olive wires and 1 half pin. The fibula is incorporated if both the tibia and fibula are incorporated into the deformity correction; otherwise, it is important to ensure that the wire fixation remains out of the fibula.

Frame extension to the foot increases stability in the distal tibial segment and creates a better environment for healing at the osteotomy site. Additionally, ankle equinus contractures are prevented or pre equinus can be treated or the ankle joint can be distracted if desired.

The foot is centered in a foot ring and secured with 5 smooth, 1.8-mm wires: 1 in the talar neck and 2 each in the calcaneal tuberosity and forefoot. The first calcaneal wire is placed from medial to posterolateral, avoiding the neurovascular structures on the medial aspect of the hindfoot, and the foot ring is secured to this wire parallel to the sole of the foot. Then, the first forefoot wire is placed proximal to the fifth metatarsal head engaging either the fifth, fourth, and third metatarsals or the fifth and first metatarsals (plantar to the second, third, and fourth metatarsals). Care is taken to avoid distorting the normal orientation of the metatarsals relative to each other.

Then, the second calcaneal wire is placed from distal–lateral to posteromedial. The second forefoot wire is placed medially to engage the first and second, and occasionally third, metatarsals. The 1.8-mm talar neck wire is then placed to avoid subtalar joint distraction. Tension is applied to the calcaneal wires and the forefoot wires, but not the talar wire.

Challenges

In our experience, the most common challenge is healing of the osteotomy after correction of the deformity. Often, juxta-articular deformities are associated with normal fibular length and do not require fibular osteotomy. The intact fibula may shield the distal tibia regenerate bone from sufficient loading to stimulate rapid consolidation. Other factors are previous injury to the bone, periosteum, and soft tissues at or near the osteotomy that delay healing. Meticulous technique in performing the osteotomies to prevent further disruption of periosteal blood supply is critical.

Initially, many patients treated with gradual correction require foot frame application for adequate stability distal to the osteotomy. As soon as there is adequate healing at the osteotomy, the foot ring is removed to improve weight bearing and hopefully accelerate healing.

Ultrasound bone stimulators (Smith Nephew) have been utilized in patients whose insurance covers this adjunct treatment. If there is poor bone formation at approximately 4 months after the osteotomy, patients are offered a bone grafting procedure to decrease time in their frames.

Complications

Routine complications with gradual correction include pin site inflammation or infection, hardware failure, decreased range of motion in the ankle and subtalar joints, and failure of the procedure to relieve pain. Direct neurovascular injury resulting from pin placement may occur despite operative caution because of posttraumatic distortion of the anatomy and scarring.

Immediate correction of a distal tibial varus may be complicated by traction injury of the posterior tibial nerve or an acute tarsal tunnel syndrome. Initial treatment consists of tarsal tunnel release. In acute corrections, a tarsal tunnel release is often performed before the osteotomy to avoid this complication, especially if there is scarring of the soft tissue medially. In gradual correction, if tarsal tunnel symptoms develop, the deformity correction can be reversed and then more slowly restarted once symptoms resolve or a tarsal tunnel release may be scheduled and then correction restarted.

General Care

Patient education is facilitated with a preoperative information packet reviewing external fixator and pin site care. Postoperative dressings remain in place for 3 to 7 days. Pin care begins as an outpatient to avoid exposing pin sites in the inpatient setting. Once sutures are removed, patients are encouraged to take a daily shower with antibacterial liquid soap and thorough water rinse to the leg and fixator. The fixator and leg are dried with a clean towel and hair dryer on a cool setting.

If the frame is extended to the foot, a walking assembly (a full ring secured to a rigid rocker walking platform) is attached to the foot ring with 4 threaded rods to suspend the foot above the full ring by 1 to 2 cm.

When early signs of pin site infection are noted, pin care is increased to twice daily, the pin site is wrapped with a gauze roll dressing, and weight bearing and physical therapy are limited. If signs and symptoms of a pin site infection do not rapidly improve, oral antibiotics are prescribed (cephalexin or clindamycin) for 5 to 7 days. A pin site infection usually begins to resolve within 24 hours of starting oral antibiotic treatment. Recalcitrant pin site infection is treated with intravenous antibiotic therapy with or without pin removal.

SUMMARY

We recommend gradual correction of distal tibia varus as most applicable for patients with severe deformities that would not be adequately corrected with acute methods. Complex deformity, compromised soft tissues, and limb shortening are, in general, better managed with this technique.

REFERENCES

1. Kettelkamp D, Hillberry B, Murrish D, et al. Degenerative arthritis of the knee secondary to fracture malunion. Clin Orthop Rel Res 1988;234:159–69.
2. Kristensen K, Klaer T, Blicher J. No arthrosis of the ankle 20 years after malaligned tibial-shaft fracture. Acta Orthop Scand 1989;60:(2):208–9.
3. McKellop H, Llinas A, Sarmiento A. Effects of tibial malalignment on the knee and ankle. Orthop Clin Nor Am 1994;25(3):415–23.
4. McKellop H, Sigholm G, Redfern F, et al. The effect of simulated fracture-angulations of the tibia on cartilage pressures in the knee joint. J Bone Joint Surg Am 1991;73A(9): 1382–91.
5. Merchant T, Dietz F, Redfern F. Long-term follow-up after fractures of the tibial and fibular shafts. J Bone Joint Surg Am 1989;71A(4):599–606.
6. Milner S, Davis T, Muir K, et al. Long-term outcome after tibial shaft fracture: is malunion important. J Bone Joint Surg Am 2002;84A(6):971–80.
7. Van Der Schoot D, Den Outer A, Bode P, et al. Degenerative changes at the knee and ankle related to malunion of tibial fractures. J Bone Joint Surg Br 1996;78B(5):722–5.
8. Puno R, Vaughan J, Stetten M, et al. Long-term effects of tibial angular malunion on the knee and ankle joints. J Orthop Trauma 1991;5:247–54.
9. Ting A, Tarr R, Sarmiento A, et al. The role of subtalar motion and ankle contact pressure changes from angular deformities of the tibia. Foot Ankle 1987;7(5):290–9.
10. Graehl P, Hersh M, Heckman J. Supramalleolar osteotomy for the treatment of symptomatic tibial malunion. J Orthop Trauma 1988;1:281–92.
11. Pearce M, Smith M, Savidge G. Supramalleolar tibial osteotomy for haemophilic arthropathy of the ankle. J Bone Joint Surg Br 1994;76B:947–50.
12. Cheng Y, Chang J, Hsu C, et al. Lower tibial osteotomy for osteoarthritis of the ankle. Kaohsiung J Med Sci 1994;10:430–7.
13. Stamatis E, Cooper P, Myerson M. Supramalleolar osteotomy for the treatment of distal tibial angular deformities and arthritis of the ankle joint. Foot Ankle Int 2003;24: 754–64.
14. Tanaka Y, Takakura Y, Hayashi K, et al. Low tibial osteotomy for varus-type osteoarthritis of the ankle. J Bone Joint Surg Br 2006;88B:909–13.
15. Pagenstert G, Hintermann B, Barg A, et al. Realignment surgery as alternative treatment of varus and valgus ankle osteoarthritis. Clin Orthop Rel Res 2007;462: 156–68.
16. Sugimoto K, Samoto N, Takakura Y, et al. Varus tilt of the tibial plafond as a factor in chronic ligament instability of the ankle. Foot Ankle Int 1997;18(7):402–5.
17. Lee W, Moon J, Lee H, et al. Alignment of ankle and hindfoot in early stage ankle osteoarthritis. Foot Ankle Int 2011;32:693–9.
18. Beaman DN, Gellman RE, Trepman E. Ankle arthritis: deformity correction and distraction arthroplasty. In: Coughlin M, Mann R, Saltzman C, editors. Surgery of the foot and ankle. 8th edition. Philadelphia (PA): Elsevier Health Sciences; 2008.

19. Beaman DN, Gellman RE, Trepman E. Foot deformity: osteotomy or arthrodesis. In: Rozbruch SR, Ilizarov GA, editors. Limb lengthening and reconstruction surgery. New York (NY): Informa Healthcare; 2007.
20. Frierson M, Ibrahim K, Boles M, et al. Distraction osteogenesis: a comparison of osteotomy techniques. Clin Orthop 1994;301:19–24.
21. Reimann I. Experimental osteoarthritis of the knee in rabbits induced by alteration of the load-bearing. Acta Orthop Scand 1973;44:496–504.

Treatment of Posttraumatic Varus Ankle Deformity with Supramalleolar Osteotomy

Markus Knupp, MD*, Lilianna Bolliger, MSc, Beat Hintermann, MD

KEYWORDS

- Varus ankle • Ankle arthritis • Supramalleolar osteotomy
- Hindfoot deformity

The most common cause of end-stage ankle arthritis is trauma.[1–3] Factors contributing to the development of posttraumatic ankle arthritis are the initial cartilage damage,[4] malreduction,[5,6] nonunion, infections, and instability.[7] In a retrospective study, Valderrabano and colleagues[1] found that 55% of patients with posttraumatic ankle arthritis presented with a varus malalignment, whereas 8% had valgus malalignment.[1] Malalignment leads to altered load distribution across the joint, interfering with normal cartilage metabolism. In young patients this interference can lead to early ankle joint arthritis, for which ankle fusion or joint replacement may not provide a lifetime solution. Therefore, supramalleolar osteotomies have gained increasing popularity to address sequelae of posttraumatic ankle joint arthritis.

This article discusses the anatomic and biomechanical properties of posttraumatic varus arthritis of the ankle joint; it also presents an overview of surgical indications and the technique of supramalleolar osteotomies for this patient population.

ANATOMY AND BIOMECHANICS

The ankle joint is part of a biomechanical chain connecting the lower leg to the foot. Therefore, hindfoot malalignment can be part of a complex deformity involving not only the lower leg but also the hindfoot, midfoot, and forefoot. In preoperative planning, two essentially different groups of varus hindfoot deformity need to be distinguished: (1) those with isolated frontal plane deformity of the hindfoot and (2) those with complex (cavo-) varus foot, which, in its severe form, is often associated with neuromuscular conditions.[8]

The ankle joint consists of three bones: the tibia, the fibula, and the talus. These bones are held together by a complex ligamentous apparatus, maintaining tight joint

The authors have no conflicts of interest to disclose.

Department of Orthopaedic Surgery, Kantonsspital Liestal, CH-4410 Liestal, Switzerland

* Corresponding author.

E-mail address: markus.knupp@ksli.ch

contact throughout the entire range of motion. Therefore, the principles of corrective osteotomies of the proximal tibia, as in high tibial osteotomies, cannot be transferred to the corrections of the ankle. In contrast to corrections of the proximal tibial articular joint surface, an isolated change of the angle of the distal tibial articular joint surface may not lead to normalization of the load distribution within the ankle joint. The reason for this failure to achieve normalization lies in the high congruency of the ankle joint: the fibula and the surrounding soft tissues may prevent the talus from following the tibia when changing the tibial articular surface (TAS) angle. As a consequence, an acute change of the TAS can lead to a paradox shift of the load transfer; medial shifts in ankles with valgus deformity and lateral shifts in ankle with varus deformity are observed.[9,10] Furthermore, ex vivo studies showed that (cavo-) varus deformities shift the load transfer not only medially but also in an anterior direction.[9,11] This aspect needs to be taken into consideration when correcting the TAS, particularly in cases with anterior extrusion of the talus from the ankle mortise.

Finally, a supramalleolar deformity leads to a static and a dynamic overload of the medial part of the ankle joint. When standing, the center of force transmission in the varus ankle is medialized, which in turn leads to medial overload. The forces on the medial side are amplified by activation of the triceps surae: because of the osseous configuration the calcaneal tuberosity is medialized. Therefore, the Achilles tendon becomes an invertor and acts as an additional deforming force on the varus hindfoot.

INDICATIONS FOR SUPRAMALLEOLAR OSTEOTOMIES

Indications for realignment surgery include corrections of malaligned ankles with medial ankle joint arthritis, corrections of malunions after distal tibia fractures, realignment before total ankle replacement, and fusion and corrections after malpositioned ankle fusions. The contraindications are end-stage arthritis, severe hindfoot instability that cannot be stabilized, severe vascular or neurologic deficiency in the affected extremity, and neuropathic disorders (eg, Charcot foot). Finally, relative contraindications that need to be considered are altered bone quality (due to medication, large cysts, and osteopenia or osteoporosis), age (>70 years), insulin-dependent diabetes, smoking, and rheumatic disease.

PREOPERATIVE PLANNING

The most important aspect of preoperative planning is assessment of the origin of the deformity. It is mandatory to separate the isolated varus deformity of the hindfoot, which is a deviation in the coronal plane, from the cavovarus foot, which essentially is a deformity involving the transverse, sagittal, and coronal planes.

Clinical Examination

Hindfoot stability needs to be assessed with routine physical examination. The range of motion of the ankle joint is captured. In arthritic joints, anterior impingement is excluded. The function of joint-crossing tendons should be tested. Finally, the Coleman block test[12] should be performed to exclude a forefoot-driven deformity.

Radiographic Examination

Radiographs that should be obtained include weight-bearing images of the entire foot, the ankle, and the tibial shaft (full-length radiographs). Unless deformity at the level of the knee joint or the femur can be excluded clinically, whole lower-limb radiographs are obtained. Furthermore, signs of stress reactions of the fifth metatarsal, medial subluxation of the talonavicular joint, and plantarflexion of the first metatarsal should be investigated. Additional hindfoot views (Saltzman view[13] or Méary view[14]) are helpful to assess the amount of coronal plane deformity. Finally, single photon-emission computed tomography (SPECT) has proved helpful for the planning of supramalleolar osteotomies, particularly in biplanar corrections.[15]

Planning of the Correction

Prior to surgery, the correction is planned on the anteroposterior and lateral view radiographs.[16] The TAS angle[17] (α; normal value, 91°–93°) is measured. The lateral view radiographs are used to distinguish between patients who present with a centered joint and those with an anterior extrusion of the talus out of the mortise. Varus feet can be corrected with a medial opening-wedge osteotomy or a lateral closing-wedge osteotomy. The decision between the lateral or medial approach is based on the amount of correction needed. In an extensive medial opening-wedge osteotomy, the fibula may restrict the amount of correction possible; therefore, deformities greater than 10° are corrected through a lateral approach (including an osteotomy of the fibula).[18] The lateral approach is also used in patients who present with a malunited fibula from a previous fracture.[16,18] To calculate and determine the size of the wedge to be inserted or removed, Warnock and colleagues[19] confirmed accuracy using the mathematical formula $\tan \alpha = H/W$, where α is the angle to be corrected, H is the wedge height in millimeters, and W is the tibial width in millimeters. An overcorrection of 2° to 5° is recommended by most investigators.[20–22]

SURGICAL TECHNIQUE

Supramalleolar osteotomies are done through a medial, anterior, or lateral approach.

Medial Approach

The medial approach is used for medial opening osteotomies. The incision lies over the distal tibia posterior to the great saphenous vein and the saphenous nerve. The tibia is exposed without stripping the periosteum. The plane of the osteotomy is determined under image intensification. A K-wire is placed from the medial to the lateral cortex, exiting the bone slightly proximally to the former growth plate or at the apex of the deformity, respecting the anatomic axis of the ankle joint (anteromedial to posterolateral[17]). Subsequently, the osteotomy is done using a wide saw blade and the correction made according to the preoperative plan. In case of anterior extrusion, the correction is carried out in a biplanar fashion, for example anterior and medial opening wedge, to improve the talar coverage in the anteroposterior direction.[21] Processed human cancellous allograft (Tutoplast, Tutogen Medical GmbH, Neunkirchen am Brand, Germany) can be used to fill the gap. Rigid plate fixation with locking screws is recommended to secure the correction (**Fig. 1**).

After completion of the tibial osteotomy, the ankle mortise is checked under image intensification. In case of joint incongruence because of inadequate length of the fibula, the fibula is osteotomized and the position and length of the fibula adjusted[23] (see **Fig. 1**).

After the supramalleolar correction, the alignment of the heel is reassessed clinically. The aim is to achieve a heel with 1° to 5° valgus. Remaining deformity must be addressed with an osteotomy of the calcaneus.[23]

Anterior Approach

The anterior approach is used in patients with altered medial/lateral soft-tissue condition and patients with significant anterior extrusion of the talus out of the

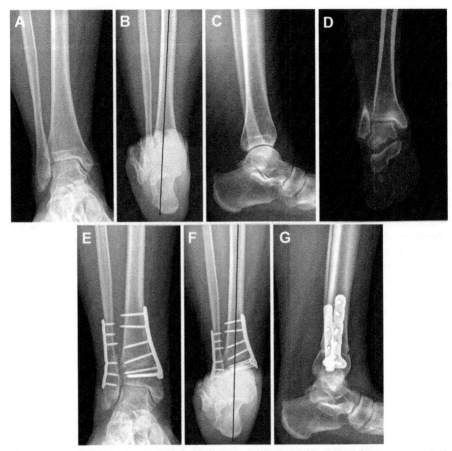

Fig. 1. A 48-year-old women with varus arthritis of the ankle joint after an operatively treated bimalleolar fracture 18 years ago. The preoperative weight-bearing images (*A–C*) show the varus malalignment in the supramalleolar area. The preoperative SPECT image (*D*) illustrates increased tracer uptake in the medial compartment of the ankle joint. Images *E, F,* and *G* were obtained 1 year postoperatively.

mortise. A longitudinal incision is made between the anterior tibial tendon and the extensor hallucis longus tendon starting from 10 cm proximal to the joint, about midway between the malleoli. The neurovascular bundle lies lateral to the incision. The anterior surface of the tibia is exposed after incising the remaining soft tissues craniocaudally. Finally, the osteotomy is carried out as described in the previous section. In the case of an anterior opening-wedge osteotomy, the talar neck is exposed and the spurs removed to compensate for the loss of dorsiflexion due to the correction of the distal tibia (**Fig. 2**).

Lateral Approach

A lateral approach is used for lateral closing-wedge osteotomies and usually includes osteotomies of both the tibia and fibula. A 10-cm longitudinal slightly curved incision is made along the anterior margin of the distal fibula. If the incision needs to be

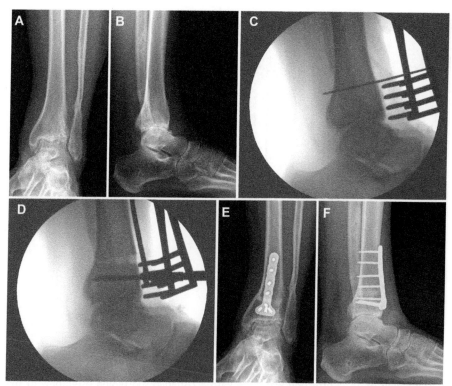

Fig. 2. A 43-year-old woman with posttraumatic arthritis 4 years after a pilon fracture. Preoperative images (*A, B*) show obliteration of the joint space anteriorly and medially. Correction was done with an anteriorly and medially opening-wedge osteotomy and a groove deepening of the talar neck (*C, D*). Images *E* and *F* were obtained 1 year postoperatively.

extended distally, it is curved ventrally to end just distal and anterior to the lateral malleolus. The fibula and the tibia are then exposed laterally. At the distal end of the incision, the anterior syndesmosis is exposed. In most cases in which a varus deformity is addressed with a lateral closing-wedge osteotomy, the fibula needs to be shortened to preserve the congruency in the ankle joint. The shortening can be done by simple bone block removal or a Z-shaped osteotomy.[16,18] K-wires are then drilled through the tibia in a converging way, and the tips should meet at the medial cortex. After the osteotomy the gap is closed, the correction is secured with a plate. Finally, the position of the fibula needs to be determined with fluoroscopy. Once the joint appears congruent, the fibula is secured with screws or a one-third tubular plate (**Fig. 3**).

POSTOPERATIVE TREATMENT

Patients are permitted to partially bear weight for 8 weeks following surgery. During this time the ankle is protected in a splint at night and a walker boot during the day. Thereafter, full weight-bearing is allowed, and physiotherapy is initiated.

RESULTS

Earlier reports have demonstrated good to excellent survival rates and improvement in clinical outcomes following supramalleolar osteotomy. Takakura and colleagues[24]

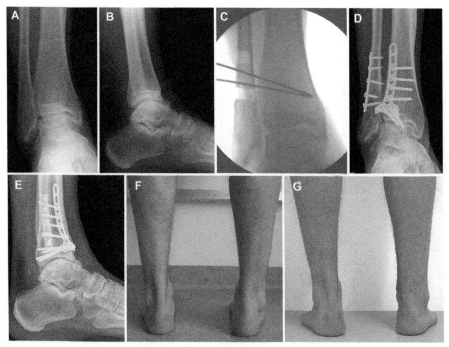

Fig. 3. A 37-year-old man with posttraumatic varus arthritis of the ankle joint 12 years after an isolated fracture of the medial malleolus. Preoperative images (*A, B*) show the varus malalignment of 15°. Correction was done with a Z-shaped shortening osteotomy of the fibula and a lateral closing-wedge osteotomy of the tibia (*C*). Images *D* and *E* were obtained 3 years postoperatively, and *F* (preoperative) and *G* (postoperative) show the clinical presentation (operated foot: right foot).

described good to excellent results in a majority of patients treated for posttraumatic varus arthritis with relief of pain and reduction of limitations in daily activities. Cheng and colleagues[21] reported on a selected series of 6 patients with posttraumatic arthritis treated with a supramalleolar osteotomy and observed good outcomes in an intermediate stage of moderate ankle arthritis. Pagenstert and colleagues[22] reported on a series of 35 patients who underwent supramalleolar osteotomies and found that total ankle replacement or ankle fusion was postponed in 91% of cases by realignment surgery. In the authors' series, they treated 29 patients (18 men, 11 women) with posttraumatic varus arthritis of the ankle joint. All of these patients had a history of a pilon or an ankle fracture. The average age of the patients was 49 years (range, 28 to 73 years). Seventeen patients were treated with a medial opening osteotomy and 12 patients with a lateral closing osteotomy. In 7 cases a biplanar osteotomy was carried out because of anterior extrusion of the talus. After a follow-up period of 45 months, the visual analogue scale for pain decreased from 4.4 (range, 0–8) to 2.6 (range, 0–7) (*P* = .003), and the American Orthopaedic Foot and Ankle Society score increased from 52 (range, 22–83) to 73 (range, 27–100) (*P*<.001). There were 10 patients who required secondary surgery: of these 10, 9 had a planned hardware removal and 1 had arthritis progression to end-stage arthritis. This patient was treated with a secondary total ankle replacement. The authors furthermore concur with earlier reports observing that an inferior result and worse outcome is found in patients with obliteration of the medial gutter.[25] This finding was, however, not statistically significant.

SUMMARY

Supramalleolar osteotomies for correction of posttraumatic varus arthritis in early and mid-stages provide good functional and clinical outcomes. However, the biomechanical behavior of the ankle joint differs from the knee, and therefore correction of the distal TAS angle alone may not provide a physiologic load transfer across the ankle joint. Osseous balancing of an arthritic varus ankle joint may require not only correction of the articular surface angle in the frontal plane but may include a biplanar correction to improve the talar coverage and a fibular osteotomy to restore ankle joint congruency.

REFERENCES

1. Valderrabano V, Horisberger M, Russell I, et al. Etiology of ankle osteoarthritis. Clin Orthop Relat Res 2009;467(7):1800–6.
2. Saltzman CL, Salamon ML, Blanchard GM, et al. Epidemiology of ankle arthritis: report of a consecutive series of 639 patients from a tertiary orthopaedic center. Iowa Orthop J 2005;25:44–6.
3. Thomas RH, Daniels TR. Ankle arthritis. J Bone Joint Surg Am 2003;85-A(5):923–36.
4. Stufkens SA, Knupp M, Horisberger M, et al. Cartilage lesions and the development of osteoarthritis after internal fixation of ankle fractures: a prospective study. J Bone Joint Surg Am 2010;92(2):279–86.
5. Thordarson DB, Motamed S, Hedman T, et al. The effect of fibular malreduction on contact pressures in an ankle fracture malunion model. J Bone Joint Surg Am 1997;79(12):1809–15.
6. Lindsjo U. Operative treatment of ankle fracture-dislocations. A follow-up study of 306/321 consecutive cases. Clin Orthop Relat Res 1985(199):28–38.
7. Harrington KD. Degenerative arthritis of the ankle secondary to long-standing lateral ligament instability. J Bone Joint Surg Am 1979;61(3):354–61.
8. Alexander IJ, Johnson KA. Assessment and management of pes cavus in Charcot-Marie-tooth disease. Clin Orthop Relat Res 1989(246):273–81.
9. Knupp M, Stufkens S, van Bergen C, et al. Effect of supramalleolar varus and valgus deformities on the tibiotalar joint: a cadaveric study. Foot Ankle Int 2011;32(6):609–15.
10. Stufkens S, van Bergen C, Blankevoort L, et al. The role of the fibula in distal tibial varus and valgus: a biomechanical study. J Bone Joint Surg Br 2011;93(9):1232–9.
11. Krause F, Windolf M, Schwieger K, et al. Ankle joint pressure in pes cavovarus. J Bone Joint Surg Br 2007;89(12):1660–5.
12. Coleman SS, Chesnut WJ. A simple test for hindfoot flexibility in the cavovarus foot. Clin Orthop Relat Res 1977(123):60–2.
13. Saltzman CL, el-Khoury GY. The hindfoot alignment view. Foot Ankle Int 1995;16(9): 572–6.
14. Morrey BF, Wiedeman GP Jr. Complications and long-term results of ankle arthrodeses following trauma. J Bone Joint Surg Am 1980;62(5):777–84.
15. Knupp M, Pagenstert GI, Barg A, et al. SPECT-CT compared with conventional imaging modalities for the assessment of the varus and valgus malaligned hindfoot. J Orthop Res 2009;27(11):1461–6.
16. Knupp M, Stufkens S, Pagenstert G, et al. Supramalleolar osteotomy for tibiotalar varus malalignment. Tech Foot Ankle Surg 2009;8(1):17–23.

17. Stiehl JB, editor. Inman's joints of the ankle. 2nd edition. Baltimore (MD): Williams and Wilkins; 1991.
18. Knupp M, Pagenstert G, Valderrabano V, et al. Osteotomies in varus malalignment of the ankle. Oper Orthop Traumatol 2008;20(3):262–73.
19. Warnock KM, Johnson BD, Wright JB, et al. Calculation of the opening wedge for a low tibial osteotomy. Foot Ankle Int 2004;25(11):778–82.
20. Takakura Y, Tanaka Y, Kumai T, et al. Low tibial osteotomy for osteoarthritis of the ankle. Results of a new operation in 18 patients. J Bone Joint Surg Br 1995;77(1):50–4.
21. Cheng YM, Huang PJ, Hong SH, et al. Low tibial osteotomy for moderate ankle arthritis. Arch Orthop Trauma Surg 2001;121(6):355–8.
22. Pagenstert GI, Hintermann B, Barg A, et al. Realignment surgery as alternative treatment of varus and valgus ankle osteoarthritis. Clin Orthop Relat Res 2007;462:156–68.
23. Knupp M, Stufkens S, Bolllger L, et al. Classification and treatment of supramalleolar deformities. Foot Ankle Int 2011;32(11):1023–31.
24. Takakura Y, Takaoka T, Tanaka Y, et al. Results of opening-wedge osteotomy for the treatment of a post-traumatic varus deformity of the ankle. J Bone Joint Surg Am 1998;80(2):213–8.
25. Tanaka Y, Takakura Y, Hayashi K, et al. Low tibial osteotomy for varus-type osteoarthritis of the ankle. J Bone Joint Surg Br 2006;88(7):909–13.

Planning Correction of the Varus Ankle Deformity with Ankle Replacement

Ken-Jin Tan, MBBS, MRCS[a],*, Mark S. Myerson, MD[b]

KEYWORDS

• Ankle • Arthritis • Deformity • Replacement • Varus

The technology and techniques of total ankle replacement have improved significantly over the last few decades. With these advances, the indications for ankle replacement have similarly expanded. Previously, ankle replacement was primarily indicated for patients with minimal coronal plane deformity. This excluded many patients from ankle replacement, because the most common pathology leading to ankle replacement is posttraumatic arthritis and this is frequently associated with a varus deformity.[1]

Increasingly, indications are beginning to include patients with coronal plane deformity. Previous recommendations have been to limit ankle replacement to a coronal deformity of less than 10°. Some reports have documented a higher failure rate in larger deformities. Coetzee[2] reported a 50% failure rate with conversion to an ankle arthrodesis in 3 years for the group of patients with preoperative varus of 20° or more. He recommended primary arthrodesis in this patient group. The latter report, however, detailed the results of treatment of the Agility prosthesis, which in our opinion is unsuitable for accurate correction of a varus deformity. With the latter prosthesis, there are only 2 sizes of the polyethylene, which is inadequate, and as we will see, is integral to the correct decision making and balancing of the ankle joint.[2] Wood and colleagues[3,4] found a higher incidence of edge loading of the polyethylene in patients with a preoperative deformity of 15° or more. They recommended that a coronal deformity of 15° or more be considered a relative contraindication to ankle replacement. The increased failure rates in these studies may be due to an inadequate correction of alignment and ligamentous balance intraoperatively, leading to edge loading of the polyethylene and premature implant failure.

The authors have nothing to disclose.

[a] Division of Foot and Ankle Surgery, University Orthopaedics Hand and Reconstructive Microsurgery Cluster, National University Hospital, 5 Lower Kent Ridge Road, NUHS Tower Block, Singapore 119074

[b] Institute for Foot and Ankle Reconstruction at Mercy, Mercy Medical Center, 301 St. Paul Place, Baltimore, MD 21202, USA

* Corresponding author.

E-mail address: tankenjin@gmail.com

With correction of alignment of the foot as well as the ankle, and ligament balance in patients with a varus deformity, it is our opinion that the outcome should not be different, even in deformities of larger magnitude. Kim and associates[5] found similar outcomes between patients who had a varus deformity of 10° to 22° and those with neutrally aligned ankles. Hobson and co-workers[6] found no difference in clinical outcomes between patients with a varus deformity of 11° to 30° and those with a varus deformity of 10° or less. They concluded that patients with a hindfoot deformity of up to 30° can expect to have similar outcomes, but cautioned that attention must be paid to obtaining a neutral alignment and a stable ankle with the ankle replacement.[6] One has to be careful, however, between the latter reference to hindfoot deformity of up to 30, and that of the ankle. Furthermore, one must distinguish between a 30°, which is intra-articular (in the ankle and associated with a defect of the distal lateral tibia), and that where there is severe tilt of the ankle with greater contracture of the deltoid ligament. This statement, therefore, depends on how the measurements of deformity are obtained.

There have been many developments and techniques that have allowed successful correction of larger varus deformities. A wider range of modularity in the polyethylene insert thickness in current implant designs has allowed a larger insert to be used during replacement to compensate for the larger gap after a neutralizing distal tibia bone cut. Various osteotomies superior to, inferior to, and at the level of the ankle joint are available for angular correction. There have also been advances in the soft-tissue releases and reconstruction to obtain ligamentous balance intraoperatively. An approach to operative planning in the varus ankle and the use of these techniques are discussed herein.

ASSESSMENT

Both a physical examination and a series of radiographs are routinely performed in the clinical assessment. The gait of the patient and the mechanical axis of the lower limbs are examined. Any deformity at the level of the knee and the presence of any varus in the tibia is noted. This is particularly important in the patient who has symptomatic knee arthritis associated with deformity, whether varus or valgus, because the correction of the latter deformity significantly affects the more distal deformity. For this reason, deformity correction must always commence proximally. Contribution to the deformity from the hindfoot and any forefoot-driven hindfoot varus is examined. The range of motion of the ankle, subtalar, and midfoot is tested. It is also important to note the soft-tissue status of the ankle region and the circulatory status. Ankle replacement in the presence of varus deformity frequently requires supplementary procedures, which may involve separate incisions. Hence, one should note the presence of scars that may complicate the surgical approach, as well as the peripheral pulses. If there is any doubt regarding the vascularity, it is advisable to perform noninvasive vascular studies before proceeding.

We routinely obtain weight-bearing radiologic studies with orthogonal views of both ankles as well as forced passive weight-bearing dorsiflexion and plantarflexion views. It is important to assess the magnitude as well as the character of the varus deformity. The varus deformity may be above the ankle joint, that is, as a result of a posttraumatic malunion of the distal tibia, at the level of the ankle joint or below the ankle joint at the level of the hindfoot or forefoot.[7] A deformity above the ankle joint is frequently due to a varus malunion of the tibia or developmental tibia vara. Deformity at the level of the ankle joint may be associated with either a congruent or incongruent joint.[4,5] A congruent joint is one in which there is intra-articular varus from erosion of the medial tibial plafond, typically from chronic, repetitive ankle instability.

This medial erosion results in an inclined plafond that is congruent to the tilted talar dome. Although the talar tilt may be quite significant in these cases, the tilt is relative to the axis of the tibia, and not the articular surface of the tibia. In incongruent varus, there is more significant talar tilt and an associated dysplastic, obliquely orientated medial malleolus. This type of deformity is often associated with chronic lateral ligamentous insufficiency and contracture of the deltoid ligament. As a result of the chronic pressure of the talus against the medial malleolus, there is gradual erosion of the latter, with an oblique inclination. The presence of any saggital plane subluxation should also be noted, because it is common to have anterior subluxation of the talus in patients with long-standing lateral ligament insufficiency. In addition, the varus deformity may also be related to a deformity of the hindfoot or forefoot level, such as in a cavovarus foot from hereditary sensory and motor neuropathy. We routinely perform a dynamic fluoroscopic evaluation of the ankle preoperatively in the office to determine if the varus deformity is mobile and reducible or rigid and fixed.

EXTRA-ARTICULAR DEFORMITY ABOVE THE ANKLE JOINT

Varus deformity above the ankle is the result of a supramalleolar varus deformity owing to a malunited tibial fracture. The best option is to correct the deformity at the level of the center of rotation of angulation, which usually corresponds with the anatomic level of the malunion. Generally in ankle replacement, it is not possible to compensate for extra-articular deformity using a larger intra-articular cut that is perpendicular to the mechanical axis. Hence, a separate osteotomy is needed to correct the supramalleolar deformity either before or during ankle replacement. The options for the osteotomy are a lateral closing wedge, medial opening wedge, or dome osteotomy. Our preference is for the opening wedge or dome osteotomy, depending on the location of the center of rotation of angulation. These 2 osteotomies do not result in loss of limb length, and allow intraoperative adjustment to a satisfactory alignment before internal fixation.

A dome osteotomy is also useful in the correction of a multiplanar deformity, in which a saggital plane deformity needs to be corrected simultaneously with the varus deformity. **Fig. 1** illustrates a case in which a dome osteotomy was done to correct for a biplanar supramalleolar deformity at the same sitting as the ankle replacement. The same anterior midline incision is used for both procedures. The planned dome osteotomy is carefully marked out using cautery at the level of the deformity, with the center of the radius of curvature of the dome at the center of rotation of angulation. The cut also needs to be planned such that there is adequate room for the tibial prosthesis and its stem after internal fixation of the osteotomy is carried out. Multiple bicortical drill holes are first made along the planned osteotomy. The drill holes are then connected with an osteotome to complete the osteotomy. The distal fragment is then manipulated in the coronal and saggital planes to correct the deformity. The osteotomy shown was then stabilized with an anterior plate and screws, allowing enough room for the subsequent implantation of the tibial component.

Although tibial osteotomy and ankle replacement can be done simultaneously, we prefer to stage the osteotomy before the ankle replacement. This allows for a more straightforward ankle replacement at the second stage. In addition, correction of the mechanical alignment can result in a marked improvement in symptoms despite radiologic features of arthritis. This may delay the subsequent replacement for some time.[8-10] We have noted that, over the past decade as we have performed supramalleolar osteotomies with increasing frequency, symptom relief has been remarkable for many patients. Although the osteotomy had often been planned as a staged procedure, that is, to correct deformity and then to proceed with replacement, for

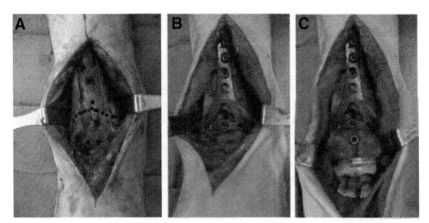

Fig. 1. Dome osteotomy and ankle replacement was done at the same time. (*A*) The osteotomy was marked with a bovie and completed. (*B*) It was first stabilized with an anterior plate which was placed superior to the tibial component. (*C*) The ankle replacement was then performed in the usual fashion.

many, the subsequent procedure was either delayed by many years, or not performed at all. For this reason, in the presence of supramalleolar varus deformity, we are inclined to perform a staged osteotomy with an opening wedge to correct alignment and shortening. However, if ankle arthritis is severe, and obviously more extensive, then the dome osteotomy is performed because this can be done simultaneously with the replacement. If the latter is chosen, however, one must be able to obtain rigid secure fixation of the osteotomy so as to facilitate early range of motion after the replacement. If there is any doubt, stage the osteotomy. It is a safe procedure, realigns the limb, and may even prolong the need for replacement. The patient presented in **Fig. 2** underwent a medial opening wedge osteotomy to correct a supramalleolar varus deformity associated with ankle arthritis. Subsequent to the osteotomy, a staged ankle replacement was then successfully performed.

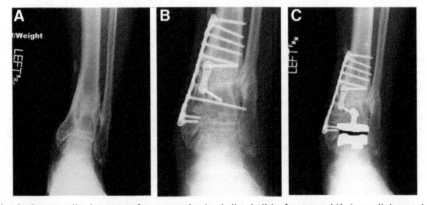

Fig. 2. Supramalleolar varus from a malunited distal tibia fracture. (*A*) A medial opening wedge osteotomy was done. (*B*) Note the neutral alignment after the osteotomy. (*C*) An ankle replacement was done subsequently.

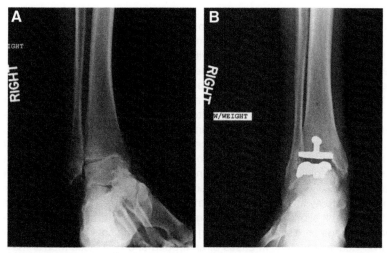

Fig. 3. (A) Preoperative AP radiograph of congruent varus ankle arthritis. Note the erosion of the tibial plafond medially. (B) Postoperative AP radiograph after ankle replacement. A neutralizing tibial cut perpendicular to the mechanical axis was made intraoperatively.

DEFORMITY AT THE LEVEL OF THE ANKLE JOINT

As discussed, deformity at the joint level may be associated with a congruent joint and intra-articular varus or an incongruent joint with a dysplastic medial malleolus. In situations of a congruent joint, a tibial cut that is perpendicular to the mechanical axis or a "neutralizing" distal tibia cut is frequently all that is needed for realignment.[5,7] This cut results in removal of a wedge of distal tibia with minimal bone resection at the eroded medial plafond and a larger resection at the lateral plafond. An appropriate thickness of polyethylene insert is chosen after realignment of the ankle, and usually the joint is stable and does not require further medial release or lateral-sided reconstruction. The latter does, however, depend on the magnitude of the deformity. Even with intra-articular varus, the deltoid may be severely contracted, and the hindfoot and forefoot deformed requiring correction. **Fig. 3** illustrates a case of a congruent varus deformity where a neutralizing tibial cut was made and an ankle replacement performed with no further adjunctive procedures.

When a significantly tilted talus with conversion of the usual vertical orientation of the medial malleolus to an oblique one is seen on preoperative radiographs, the surgeon should be prepared for a more complicated procedure. These cases usually have underlying chronic lateral ligamentous instability and require additional procedures to balance the ankle. The correction should begin with a thorough debridement of the lateral gutter. Osteophytes and debris in the lateral gutter are common findings in underlying chronic lateral instability. This prevents rotation of the talus into a neutral alignment; aggressive debridement of the gutter is necessary. A second lateral incision just posterior to the fibula can be used to debride any osteophytes over the lateral malleolus and within the lateral gutter. This incision can be extended to isolate the peroneus brevis tendon for a lateral ankle stabilization, which is not uncommon in such cases.

After the distal tibia cut is made perpendicular to the mechanical axis, we place 2 laminar spreaders into the joint space medially and laterally. If the ankle is balanced, the talar dome should now be parallel to the cut surface of the distal tibia both clinically and fluoroscopically. If the talar dome is still in varus tilt, the articular gaps is asymmetric, with a smaller medial gap. This maneuver indicates that the medial structures (the deltoid ligament, posteromedial capsule, and posterior tibial tendon) are tight and the next step is to proceed with a medial sided release. There are various alternatives for the medial release. The deep deltoid may be released directly.[6] The deep deltoid may also be released subperiosteally by sliding an osteotome or knife down the medial border of talus.[11] Some authors also perform releases of the tibialis posterior tendon[6] or the superficial deltoid.[4,11] We have used a deltoid release commonly in the past, but have not found this to be completely reliable; in some cases, it may cause medial instability. The release of the deltoid may also devascularize a portion of the talus, depending on the manner in which the deltoid is cut, because this may disturb the deltoid branch of the tibial artery. Recently, therefore, we have preferably performed the medial release using a lengthening medial malleolus osteotomy as described by Doets and colleagues[12] and have found this to be quite reliable. It allows a controlled lengthening of the medial side of the ankle and has the advantage of reliable bony healing compared with soft-tissue releases, which may never heal adequately. In cases of an eroded and dysplastic medial malleolus, the osteotomy can also be used to restore the morphology of the mortise to better capture the talus.

We start by inserting a guide pin obliquely from the proximal aspect of the medial malleolus, aiming toward the medial shoulder of the mortise. This is checked fluoroscopically and the osteotomy is then marked out with cautery. An oscillating saw is used to make the cut along the planned osteotomy. The medial malleolus is then allowed to slide distally and provisionally fixed with K-wires. The amount of distal excursion is determined by the amount of medial contracture and is usually about 5 mm. Although Doets and co-workers did not recommend fixation of the osteotomy, we routinely fix the osteotomy with cannulated screws and have found this to be quite reliable. The screws need to be placed such that they avoid the base plate and the proximal stem of the tibial component. Once the prosthesis is in place, the osteotomy is stabilized. It is then important to recheck the profile of the medial gutter to ensure that there is no impinging bone against the prosthesis. This may occur because of the change in the direction of the medial malleolus, and depends on the orientation of the osteotomy. If the osteotomy is made from proximal and medial to distal and lateral, the malleolus slides slightly toward the talus. Any impinging bone needs to be removed, is best done with a saw, and can be shaved off either the talus or the medial malleolus (**Fig. 4**). Although screws are used, one could also consider the use of an antiglide plate placed on the distal medial tibia to capture the osteotomy. We have no experience with this technique, but further analysis may prove that this method of fixation permits earlier mobilization and rehabilitation.

In cases of more severe varus tilt of the talus with a significantly dysplastic medial malleolus and incongruent joint, a useful alternative osteotomy is the medial tibial plafondplasty.[13,14] Such deformities cannot be adequately treated with a standard supramalleolar osteotomy (dome or opening wedge), because this does not address the erosion of the medial plafond and the oblique orientation of the medial malleolus. Tanaka and associates[10] reported poor results with low tibial osteotomy in cases associated with loss of joint space at the medial talar dome. The plafondplasty is able to address these issues. This is done as a separate, staged procedure before the ankle replacement and is a powerful osteotomy for restoring the congruency of the ankle joint and the profile of the mortise. The plafondplasty is performed through a medial incision along the subcutaneous border of the tibia. A guide pin is inserted in the medial tibia and inserted to exit at a point in the plafond just medial to the midpoint

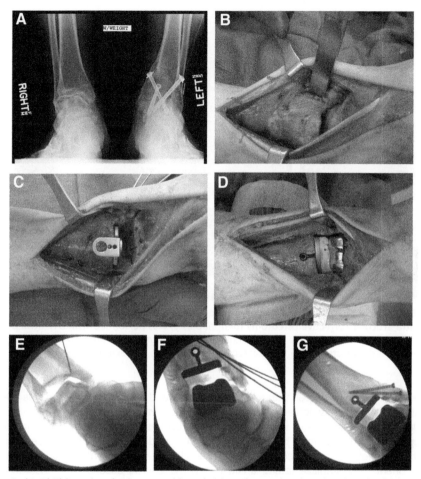

Fig. 4. (*A–D*) This patient had varus ankle arthritis and a previously arthrodesed ankle on the contralateral side. The osteotomy was planned with a K-wire, marked with a bovie, and made with an oscillating saw. A periosteal elevator was inserted to ensure that the osteotomy was complete. Wires were used for provisional stabilization after distal translation of the malleolus with the tibial trial in situ. (*D*) Neutral alignment after the definitive components were implanted. (*E–G*) Another case of medial malleolar osteotomy demonstrating intraoperative fluoroscopy views. The plane of osteotomy is planned with a K-wire and completed; then, it was provisionally fixed with cannulated wires. The wires were replaced with cannulated screws after the prosthesis was implanted.

where the articular erosion ends. This acts as a guide for the planned osteotomy. Three additional K-wires are then inserted under fluoroscopic guidance parallel to and 6 mm above the joint line in the subchondral bone of the distal tibia. These K-wires act to prevent violation of the articular surface by the oscillating saw used for the osteotomy. An oscillating saw is used to make the osteotomy to the level of the 3 K-wires. Then, a broad osteotome is inserted to hinge open the osteotomy. The medial malleolar fragment is hinged downward to restore a more normal morphology of the ankle mortise. It is important to debride the lateral gutter to facilitate realignment and also to obtain lateral sided stability, which may require an additional, lateral-sided reconstruction. The

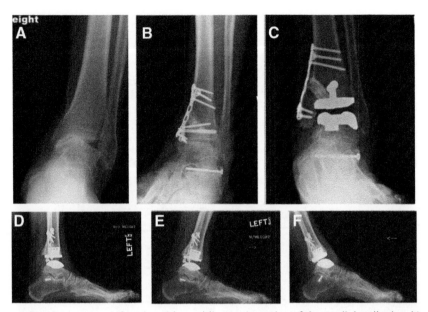

Fig. 5. Significant varus deformity with an oblique orientation of the medial malleolus. (*A–C*) An intra-articular corrective osteotomy (plafondplasty) was performed with a neutral post-operative alignment. An ankle replacement was subsequently performed. (*D–F*) Good range of motion is demonstrated on the postreplacement flexion and extension views.

osteotomy is then held open with a laminar spreader and packed tightly with bone graft. Fixation can be reliably achieved with a plate and screws (**Fig. 5**).

Once the medial side of the ankle has been addressed, the presence of lateral-sided ligament laxity must be considered. If the medial side has been adequately released (whether with osteotomy or deltoid release), a large enough polyethylene component may stabilize lateral ankle instability. This is assessed by inserting 2 laminar spreaders that are reinserted into the joint space and the presence of any lateral-sided laxity is noted, which requires a lateral-sided reconstruction. This can only be performed once the prosthesis has been inserted. A Brostrom-type technique alone is not likely to be adequate to stabilize the ankle, because the lateral ligamentous complex is usually severely attenuated. Coetzee[2] described passing the split peroneus brevis through a subcutaneous tunnel into the anterior incision and securing it with a staple into the anterolateral distal tibia. We have described using a split peroneus brevis tendon and routing this under a 2-hole plate placed over the fibula as a modified Evans type of reconstruction. The lateral incision used for debridement of the lateral gutter is extended proximally and the peroneal tendons identified. The peroneus brevis is split longitudinally and the anterior half of the peroneus brevis is harvested proximally and left intact distally. This anterior slip is then passed through an oblique 4.5-mm drill hole in the lateral malleolus, tensioned, and fixed to the fibula shaft using a 2-hole plate using compression screws. If the tendon slip is adequately tensioned, the ankle joint is balanced and in neutral alignment and has no gapping or instability on range of motion of the prosthesis (**Fig. 6**).

If there is any additional tendency for hindfoot varus, it is necessary to assess the foot for any hindfoot varus or a plantarflexed first ray. For a successful result, these also need to be corrected.

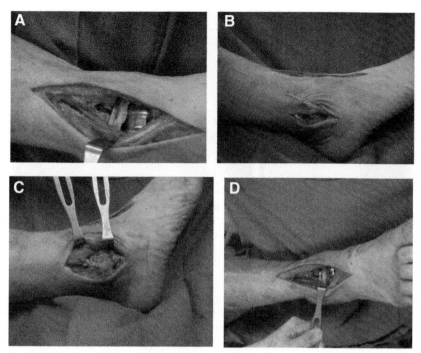

Fig. 6. (*A*) Alignment of the ankle replacement is shown intraoperatively. Note the varus tilt of the talar component with asymmetric gaps due to ligament imbalance. (*B*) The peroneus brevis tendon, which was harvested from a separate lateral incision. (*C*) The tendon was passed through an oblique drill hole starting from the tip of the lateral malleolus and exiting at the posterior cortex of the fibula shaft proximally. The tendon was then stabilized with a 2-hole compression plate onto the fibula shaft. (*D*) Note the neutral alignment of the ankle replacement after the ligament reconstruction. The gaps are symmetric.

DEFORMITY DISTAL TO THE ANKLE JOINT

Residual hindfoot or forefoot varus can cause asymmetric loading of the polyethylene, resulting in premature failure. This can occur even if the ankle replacement has been implanted with the joint line perpendicular to the mechanical axis. Thus, it is critical to assess the hindfoot and forefoot for any varus both preoperatively as well as intraoperatively, once the prosthesis has been inserted.

The hindfoot varus may originate from the heel or from an imbalance of forces acting on the hindfoot, such as a contracted tibialis posterior tendon, deficient peroneus brevis, or a medially displaced Achilles tendon. If the heel is in varus after an ankle replacement has been implanted, a simple realignment that can be performed is a lateralizing calcaneal osteotomy. A lateral incision just posterior to the peroneal tendons is made, and this is deepened to the lateral wall of the calcaneum, preserving the sural nerve in the subcutaneous layer. An oblique osteotomy of the calcaneal tuberosity is then made with a broad oscillating saw, carefully perforating the medial cortex. The osteotomy is then distracted with a laminar spreader to mobilize the tuberosity. The tuberosity is then shifted laterally by about 8 to 10 mm, depending on the amount of preexisting varus deformity. If a greater amount of correction is needed, a laterally based closing wedge may also be added. We typically stabilize the osteotomy with 2 cannulated partially threaded cancellous screws (**Fig. 7**).

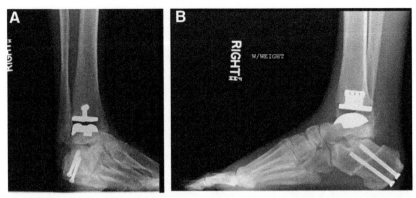

Fig. 7. (A, B) A case of varus ankle arthritis where there was a tendency for hindfoot varus after implantation of the ankle replacement. A lateralizing calcaneal osteotomy was used to neutralize the hindfoot alignment. This was stabilized with 2 partially threaded cannulated screws at the time of surgery.

A plantarflexed first ray may also contribute to hindfoot varus. This is usually associated with a cavovarus deformity of the foot. A variety of procedures may need to be done, depending on the character of the deformity, extent of muscle imbalance, and rigidity of the cavovarus deformity. A dorsiflexion osteotomy of the first ray or dorsiflexion arthrodesis at the first tarsometatarsal joint may be required, together with a transfer of the peroneus longus to the peroneus brevis. In general, in such cases, osteotomies and/or fusions with rebalancing of the foot are required in addition to the ankle replacement (**Fig. 8**). In these situations, we prefer to stage the ankle replacement after correction of the foot. This gives adequate time for the additional incisions, osteotomies, and fusions to heal first. In addition, the rehabilitation of the 2 procedures may differ and may hamper the early weight-bearing and range-of-motion exercise program we routinely use for rehabilitation after an ankle replacement.

COMBINED DEFORMITIES

Combined deformities present a complex problem. In such cases, our preference is to correct the associated deformities, followed by a staged ankle replacement. With regard to the sequence of correction, the supramalleolar deformities are corrected first, followed by correction of the hindfoot and forefoot varus. Ligamentous reconstruction may also be addressed at this stage. Finally, after healing of the reconstructions and resumption of ambulation and range of motion in the ankle, a staged ankle replacement is performed.

LIMITS TO CORRECTION OF VARUS DEFORMITY

Currently, there is no universal agreement as to an absolute limit of varus deformity that can or should be corrected with ankle replacement. What is clear is that, if a neutrally aligned and balanced ankle is not obtained after ankle replacement, the joint is prone to edge loading of the polyethylene and early failure. Doets and colleagues[12] had originally suggested that a preoperative varus or valgus deformity of more than 10° be an absolute contraindication to ankle arthroplasty. In their series of ankle replacements in inflammatory joint disease, no adjunctive procedures for the correction of deformity were described. Ankles that had a preoperative coronal deformity of

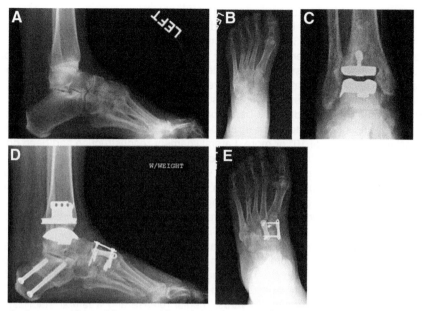

Fig. 8. Cavovarus foot with varus ankle arthritis. (*A–E*) The foot was corrected with a midfoot osteotomy and arthrodesis as well as a lateralizing calcaneal osteotomy. Ankle replacement was subsequently performed.

more than 10° had only a 48% survival rate at 8 years compared with a 90% survival rate for neutrally aligned ankles. Wood and Deakin[3] showed that a persistent coronal deformity postoperatively significantly affected outcome. In this series of 200 ankle replacements, 9 ankles showed this appearance and out of the 9, 3 ankles had severe pain requiring a revision to an arthrodesis and another 3 had aching pain and underwent a secondary procedure in an attempt to correct alignment that was only partially successful. Although another 3 were asymptomatic and left alone, the follow-up in this series was mid term at 46 months and it is possible that these would also end in premature failure. In their series, Wood and Deakin[3] also analyzed the effect of preoperative ankle alignment on outcome. They found that out of the 9 ankles that had postoperative edge loading, 7 had a preoperative deformity of more than 15°. This made up 18% of the 39 ankles that had a preoperative deformity of more than 15°. Consequently, they recommended that a deformity of more than 15° be considered a relative contraindication to ankle replacement. Coetzee[2] also cautioned against performing ankle replacement in ankles with a preoperative varus of more than 20°. In his series, this population had a 50% failure rate with conversion to an ankle arthrodesis within 3 years.

With the use of adjunctive procedures to obtain a neutrally aligned ankle replacement, recently published results have been more encouraging. Hintermann and associates[15] reported on the results of 122 ankle replacements, in which 43 additional procedures were done simultaneously. In all, 82% had good to excellent results after a mean follow-up of 18.9 months, with a revision rate of 6.6%.

Hobson and colleagues[6] compared the results of ankles with preoperative coronal deformity of 10° or less with those with a deformity of 11° to 30°. In this series, adjunctive procedures to obtain a neutral alignment included debridement of the gutters, release of the deltoid, lengthening of the tibialis posterior, calcaneal osteotomy, and subtalar fusion. No lateral-sided stabilization was carried out intraoperatively. In their series of 123 ankles with a mean follow-up of 4 years, they found no difference in the postoperative range of motion or complications between both groups. However, the most common mode of failure in both groups was postoperative instability. When a lateral ligament reconstruction was done in an attempt to address this at a later time, this was not successful in all cases.

Haskell and Mann[4] studied the behavior of the coronal plane alignment in the 2 years after an ankle replacement in 86 patients, 35 of whom had a preoperative coronal malalignment of 10° or more. Lateral ligament reconstruction had been done in 6 patients and superficial deltoid release in 4. They found that the weight-bearing axis of ankles with preoperative deformity was consistently improved toward neutral postoperatively and found no changes in alignment over the subsequent 2 years. However, patients with preoperative incongruent joints were 10 times more likely to develop edge loading on follow-up radiographs compared with those with congruent joints.

This is in contrast with the study by Kim and associates,[5] which found no significant difference in short-term outcomes between congruent and incongruent varus groups. Kim and colleagues approached the correction of the varus deformity in a stepwise fashion, addressing both realignment and ligamentous balance. They performed a neutralizing tibial cut in congruent varus, medial release and a lateral stabilization procedure in more severe cases, and combined these with a calcaneal osteotomy and/or a dorsiflexion osteotomy of the first metatarsal if needed. They reported on the results comparing 23 ankles with a preoperative varus of between 10° and 28° to 22 ankles with neutral alignment. At a mean follow-up of 27 months, there was no difference in clinical and radiologic outcome between the 2 groups, nor was there any difference in the results between the congruent and incongruent varus deformities.

SUMMARY

Ankle replacement in the presence of a varus deformity is an evolving field. Although the initial results were disappointing, numerous advances in the understanding of the condition and operative techniques have been made. More recent reports show good short-term results, especially when adjunctive procedures are combined, not only to achieve a neutral alignment but also the restore lateral ligamentous stability. As a result, it is possible to correct varus deformities of 20° or more with ankle replacement. It is likely that, with a reliable correction of alignment and balance, that the long-term results of ankle replacement in significant varus deformity will be promising.

REFERENCES

1. Valderrabano V, Horisberger M, Russell I, et al. Etiology of ankle osteoarthritis. Clin Orthop Relat Res 2009;467:1800–6.
2. Coetzee, JC. Surgical strategies: lateral ligament reconstruction as part of the management of varus ankle deformity with ankle replacement. Foot Ankle Int 2010;31:267–74.
3. Wood, PL, Deakin S. Total ankle replacement: the results in 200 ankles. J Bone Joint Surg [Br] 2003;85–B:334–41.
4. Haskell A, Mann RA. Ankle arthroplasty with preoperative coronal plane deformity. Clin Orthop Rel Res 2004;424:98–103.
5. Kim BS, Choi WJ, Kim YS, et al. Total ankle replacement in moderate to severe varus deformity of the ankle. J Bone Joint Surg [Br] 2009;91–B:1183–90.

6. Hobson SA, Karantana A, Dhar S. Total ankle replacement in patients with significant pre-operative deformity of the hindfoot. J Bone Join Surg [Br] 2009;91–B:481–86.
7. Ryssman D, Myerson MS. Surgical strategies: the management of varus ankle deformity with joint replacement. Foot Ankle Int 2011;32:217–24.
8. Pagenstert GI, Hintermann B, Barg A, et al. Realignment surgery as alternative treatment of varus and valgus ankle osteoarthritis. Clin Orthop Relat Res 2007;462: 156–8.
9. Stamatis ED, Cooper PS, Myerson MS. Supramalleolar osteotomy for the treatment of distal tibial angular deformities and arthritis of the ankle joint. Foot Ankle Int 2003;24: 754–64.
10. Tanaka Y, Takakura Y, Hayashi K, et al. Low tibia osteotomy for varus-type osteoarthritis of the ankle. J Bone Joint Surg [Br] 2006;88–B:909–13.
11. Coetzee JC. Management of varus or valgus ankle deformity with ankle replacement. Foot Ankle Clin North Am 2008;13:509 –20.
12. Doets HC, van der Plaat LW, Klein, JP. Medial malleolar osteotomy for the correction of varus deformity during total ankle arthroplasty: results in 15 ankles. Foot Ankle Int 2008;29:171–7.
13. Mann H, Filippi J, Myerson MS. Results of intra-articular opening wedge osteotomy of the medial malleolus (plafond-plasty) for the treatment of intra-articular varus ankle arthritis and ankle instability. AOFAS, Annual summer meeting. Washington, DC, 2010.
14. Myerson MS, Mann H. The use of plafondplasty intra-articular osteotomy to correct varus deformity of the ankle joint. AOFAS, Annual summer meeting. Washington, DC, 2010.
15. Hintermann B, Valderrabano V, Dereymaeker G, et al. The Hintegra ankle: rationale and short-term results of 122 consecutive ankles. Clin Orthop 2004;424:57–68.

Varus Hindfoot Deformity After Talar Fracture

James A. Sproule, MB, BAO, BCh, MCh, FRCSI, FRCS (Tr & Orth)[a,*],
Mark A. Glazebrook, MD, MSc, PhD, FRCSC[a],
Alastair S. Younger, MD, ChB, FRCSC[b]

KEYWORDS

• Talus • Fracture • Malunion • Arthrosis • Reconstruction
• Arthrodesis

The unique anatomy of the talus contributing to three important joints makes its integrity and joint congruency crucial for normal foot function.[1,2] Consequently, posttraumatic malalignment of the talus with resultant deformity almost invariably leads to painful functional impairment.

Malunion after inaccurate reduction of talar neck fractures has a reported incidence as high as 47%, with varus malunion occurring most frequently, particularly after closed reduction of displaced Hawkins type II fractures.[1–6] Typical features of malunited talar neck fractures include varus malalignment of the talar neck that causes shortening and deformity of the medial column. The foot adopts a hindfoot varus and internal rotation attitude with concurrent forefoot adduction. Range of motion in the peritalar articulations is compromised, particularly eversion in the subtalar joint.[1,2,7] Nonunion is a less common complication, with an overall reported incidence of 2.5%–3.3% of talar neck fractures.[4,6,8,9] However, nonunion is observed in up to 12% of cases of inadequately treated Hawkins type III fractures.[6] The issue with nonunion is persisting fracture fragment mobility with resultant deformity, joint incongruity, and susceptibility to posttraumatic arthritis.

Salvage procedures after talar malunions and nonunions with joint involvement, resulting in symptomatic posttraumatic arthritis, include reorientating arthrodeses of the ankle, subtalar, or talonavicular joints; triple arthrodesis; total ankle arthroplasty (TAA); and tibiotalocalcaneal arthrodesis with or without astragalectomy.[1,2,6,9–12] Although these interventions frequently effect a substantial improvement, none of them will restore normal foot function.

[a] Department of Orthopaedic Surgery, QEII Health Sciences Centre, Halifax Infirmary, 1796 Summer Street, Halifax NS, B3H 3A7, Canada
[b] Department of Orthopaedics, University of British Columbia, British Columbia's Foot and Ankle Clinic, St. Pauls Hospital, 560 1144 Burrard Street, Vancouver, BC, V6Z 2A5, Canada
* Corresponding author.
E-mail address: sproulejames@hotmail.com

Foot Ankle Clin N Am 17 (2012) 117–125
doi:10.1016/j.fcl.2011.11.009
1083-7515/12/$ – see front matter © 2012 Elsevier Inc. All rights reserved.

Secondary anatomic reconstruction, with preservation of the joints, thus seems to be a worthwhile alternative if the joint cartilage is still viable and no talar collapse or infection has occurred.[1,2,6] Near-normal foot function can be restored in cases of residual deformity after overlooked or improperly treated talar neck fractures with axial malalignment and joint incongruity.

VARUS MALALIGNMENT OF THE TALAR NECK—EFFECT ON THE FOOT

Talar neck fractures are often associated with medial comminution—with forced supination of the hindfoot, the talar neck encounters and impacts against the medial malleolus, leading to medial neck comminution and rotatory displacement of the head.[4] Varus malalignment results from inadequate reduction because of limited medial exposure or fixation with lag screws. It occurs most frequently in Hawkins type II fractures that have been treated in a closed manner.[1-6] Varus malunion causes shortening of the medial column, hindfoot varus and internal rotation, forefoot adduction, and loss of subtalar and midtarsal motion, particularly subtalar eversion.[1,2,7]

At heel strike, when the hindfoot is in valgus the forefoot is supple, because the talonavicular and calcaneocuboid joints are parallel. This property increases the mobility of these joints and allows them to adapt to undulating terrain. As the weight of the body shifts forward and the heel rises, the hindfoot inverts and the midtarsal axes lose their parallel relationship, resulting in a decrease in the mobility of the midtarsal joints. The midfoot becomes a rigid lever arm in preparation for toe-off. It is possible that the varus and internally rotated position attained by the hindfoot following varus malalignment of the talar neck decreases the mobility of the midtarsal joints and interferes with the normal reciprocal relationship between the hindfoot and midfoot.[7]

The degree of displacement at the talar neck that can result in increased morbidity and the guidelines to define an acceptable reduction have been variably described.[1,2,5-7,9,10,13] Because treatment of talar neck malunion is difficult, prevention of this complication is important. In the past, an acceptable reduction of the talar neck was considered to be less than 5 mm of displacement, and 5° of varus. However, biomechanical investigations on cadaveric specimens with pressure-sensitive film revealed that simulated malalignment of only 2 mm at the talar neck resulted in significant load redistribution between the posterior, medial, and anterior facets of the subtalar joint. These small displacements are likely critical and can lead to altered subtalar joint mechanics and arthritis.[1,2,5-7,13] Therefore, the more anatomic the reduction of the talar neck, the less the subtalar motion and position of the foot are adversely affected.

PATIENT ASSESSMENT

Indications for surgical intervention are intractable pain, gait disturbance, and significant functional incapacity.[2] A full history of the mechanism of injury, associated injuries, and interventions to date, including any early or late complications, are noted.

Pertinent physical findings are documented. Typically, patients will have a shortened medial column with hindfoot varus and internal rotation and forefoot adduction (**Fig. 1**). There is restricted range of motion in the subtalar and midtarsal joints. The overall presentation is that of a painful, rigid, cavovarus foot. This configuration impacts negatively on gait, because excessive weight-bearing on the lateral border of the foot results in lateral overload with inevitable painful callus formation. A neurovascular examination is performed, and the status of the overlying integument, including previous incisions, should be observed.

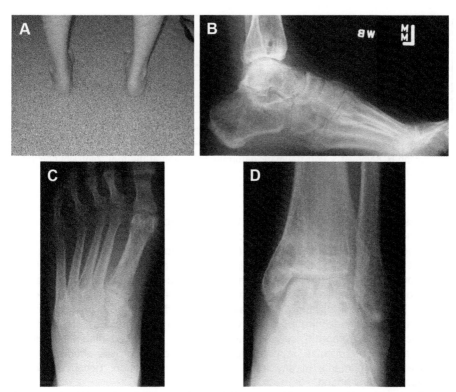

Fig. 1. Malposition of a displaced talar neck fracture. This 25-year-old patient fell from a balcony 3 years prior to assessment. He was treated nonoperatively because the consulting surgeon did not believe the deformity merited reduction. However, the patient had ongoing hindfoot varus and discomfort in the subtalar joint. (A) The hindfoot varus from behind on the left side. (B–D) The united talar neck fracture with some dorsal displacement of the talar neck, internal rotation of the forefoot on the anteroposterior (AP) view of the foot, and subtle medial translation of the subtalar joint on the AP view of the ankle indexed by the lateral step between the talus and calcaneus.

Routine leucocyte count, erythrocyte sedimentation rate, and C-reactive protein should be obtained for all patients to rule out infection.[2,9] Weight-bearing anteroposterior, dorsoplantar, and lateral radiographs of the foot and ankle, including a hindfoot alignment view of both feet, are obtained. Radiographic evidence of posttraumatic arthritis, avascular necrosis (AVN), osseous displacement, joint incongruity, and quality of bone stock are assessed. A special oblique view of the talar neck, described by Canale and Kelly,[10] provides the best evaluation of talar neck angulation and shortening, which is not appreciable on routine radiographs. The view is acquired by placing the ankle in maximum plantarflexion, pronating the foot 15°, and angling the x-ray tube 75° from the horizontal with the beam directed cephalad. Computed tomography (CT) scans should be sought in all cases to assess joint incongruities and degeneration and to permit precise preoperative planning.[2,6,14–16]

If these investigations are suggestive of AVN, its presence and extent can be further elucidated with magnetic resonance imaging (MRI). MRI can also be used to evaluate the magnitude of chondral damage that is present. AVN is considered to be partial if less than one-third of the talar body is involved and complete if greater than one-third

Table 1	
Classification of posttraumatic talar deformity	
Type	Findings
I	Malunion with joint displacement
II	Nonunion with joint displacement
III	Types I/II with partial AVN
IV	Types I/II with complete AVN
V	Types I/II with septic AVN

From Zwipp H, Rammelt S. Post-traumatic deformity correction at the foot. Zentralbl Chir 2003; 128(3):219.

of the talar body is affected, leading to talar collapse. A classification for talar deformities has been previously proposed (Table 1).[17]

In types I to III deformity, delayed anatomic reconstruction of the talus, with adjacent joint preservation, is justified in compliant, active patients with sufficient bone stock. Types I to III deformities with symptomatic posttraumatic arthritis can be salvaged with axial realignment and fusion, with preservation of either the ankle or subtalar joints where possible. On occasion, the final decision to reconstruct or fuse a joint can only be made intraoperatively while assessing the cartilage status. Patients with background comorbidities, for example poorly controlled diabetes mellitus, peripheral vascular disease, immune deficiency, or osteoporosis, should be duly cautioned on the merits of any form of surgical intervention, because perilous complications may ensue.

In patients with complete AVN and collapse of the talar body (type IV deformities), the choice operation is usually a tibiotalocalcaneal fusion with autologous bone grafting, after excision of residual necrotic bone. In the presence of sepsis (type V deformities), repeated debridement of infected, necrotic bone consistently culminates in subtotal talectomy, although in some cases the talar head, and thus the talonavicular joint, may be preserved.[2,6]

The rest of this article concentrates on posttraumatic type I and II talar deformities with no marked evidence of AVN, collapse, or sepsis.

PRIMARY ANATOMIC REDUCTION AND INTERNAL FIXATION

As alluded to previously, treatment of talar neck malunion is difficult. Thus, prevention of this complication is important in the definitive treatment of talar neck fractures in the primary setting. Displaced fractures should be accurately reduced and internally fixed.[1–6,18–29] The more anatomic the reduction of talar neck fractures, the less adverse the impact on subtalar and midtarsal motion and on the position of the foot.[7]

Medial neck comminution or impaction is often underestimated and is a major contributing factor to varus malunion.[1–6,9,18,20,21] A number of measures have been recommended to counter such an occurrence. A dual incision approach using both a medial and anterolateral or oblique lateral (Ollier) incision may permit a more optimal assessment of the accuracy of fracture reduction and fixation.[4,6,8,20,21] However, surgical exposure can contribute to circulatory compromise of the talus.[4,6,21,30] Care must be taken to avoid stripping of the dorsal neck vessels and to preserve the deltoid branches entering at the level of the deep deltoid ligament. A wide enough skin bridge must also be maintained between the two incisions to avoid skin necrosis. Lag screws can be used for fixation of talar neck fractures but in the presence of medial neck comminution can result in neck shortening and varus malalignment when the fracture is compressed. In such cases the use of fully threaded cannulated cancellous screws in a neutralization (noncompression) mode is preferable. Bone graft is occasionally necessary to make up for large impaction defects of the medial talar neck.[4,19–21] Minifragment (2 mm–2.7 mm) plating techniques can be especially helpful to maintain length of the medial column and can buttress the fracture as well as any bone graft that is added to the fracture gap.[19–21,31]

SECONDARY ANATOMIC RECONSTRUCTION

In cases of talar neck nonunions and malunions, consideration of the peritalar articulations should be undertaken. Secondary anatomic reconstruction seems attractive in young, compliant patients with adequate bone stock if the joint cartilage is still viable and no talar collapse or infection has occurred.[2,6,9]

Surgery is performed under tourniquet control, and the iliac crest is draped free to allow access for autologous bone grafting when indicated. In most instances a dual approach is used. The anteromedial approach permits exposure of the ankle and talonavicular joints, and an additional anterolateral or oblique lateral (Ollier) approach allows visualization of the subtalar joint. A medial malleolar osteotomy may be warranted when the fracture extends into the talar body.

It is important to respect the residual vascularity of the talus. Extensive soft-tissue dissection of the dorsum of the talar neck and at the tip of the medial malleolus needs to be avoided. Access to joints can be optimized by arthrodiastasis via a femoral distractor placed between the tibia and calcaneus (**Fig. 2**). The original fracture through the talar neck or body is exposed. Resection of fibrous pseudoarthrosis and sclerotic bone to viable, cancellous bone is performed in the case of nonunions. When a varus malunion exists, a correctional osteotomy is made along the former fracture plane. The viability of the cartilage at the ankle and subtalar and talonavicular joints is assessed by thorough inspection. Loose, nonviable fragments are excised. Smaller chondral lesions may be treated with debridement and microfracture. However, if extensive full-thickness chondral defects are noted, arthrodesis should be considered after correction of the deformity. The vascularity of the talar body may also be checked with the tourniquet released. Avascular areas may benefit from subchondral drilling to encourage bone revitalization.[2]

Mobilized fragments are reduced anatomically. Cancellous bone grafting is performed in preexisting nonunions to maintain the length of the medial talar neck after resection of sclerotic bone. A wedge-shaped autologous tricortical iliac crest graft is harvested and used for axial correction where an opening wedge osteotomy of the talar neck is performed for varus malunion. After anatomic reconstruction, definitive stable osteosynthesis is carried out using a variety of potential fixation techniques. Surgical restoration of the anatomic shape of the talus after malunion or nonunion of a displaced neck or body fracture with preservation of the essential joints has been reported only occasionally. Monroe and Manoli[5] described a case of malunion of the talar neck after a Hawkins type II fracture in a 34-year-old man after nonoperative treatment. This nonunion was successfully corrected with an osteotomy of the talar neck, insertion of a tricortical iliac crest bone graft, and stable internal fixation. The osteotomy healed uneventfully, with no evidence of AVN. The deformity correction was maintained. Rammelt and colleagues[1] reported on 10 patients with painful malunions or nonunions who were treated over an 8-year period with secondary anatomic reconstruction at a mean of 1 year after sustaining displaced talar body or

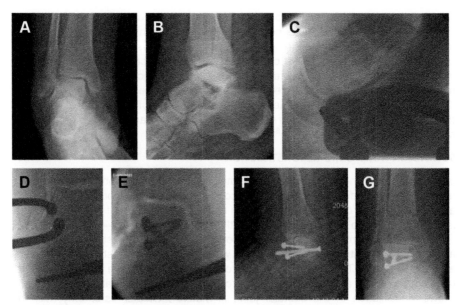

Fig. 2. A 74-year-old woman with a talar neck fracture that was missed at the time of injury. The foot was fixed in an internally rotated position with subluxation of the subtalar joint. (*A, B*) Radiographs performed at the time of presentation. (*C–E*) Reduction of the partial union using external fixation and ankle arthroscopy to identify the fracture site from within the ankle and mobilization of the fracture site arthroscopically to prevent loss of blood supply to the talus. Percutaneous reduction and fixation was used. (*F, G*) Follow-up radiographs 1 year after surgery.

neck fractures. Correction was by an osteotomy through the malunited fracture or removal of the pseudoarthrosis. Internal fixation was achieved with screws and additional bone grafting if necessary. Uneventful solid union was obtained in all cases, with no signs of the development or progression of AVN. At a mean of 4 years after reconstruction, all patients were satisfied with the result except for 1 patient who required ankle fusion. The mean American Orthopaedic Foot and Ankle Society Ankle Hindfoot Score increased from 38 to 86 ($P<.001$). The investigators concluded that secondary anatomic reconstruction with joint preservation leads to considerable functional improvement in painful talar malunions and nonunions.[1] Huang and Cheng[3] reported on 9 patients who underwent delayed surgical treatment for neglected or malreduced talar fractures at time intervals postinjury from 4 weeks to 4 years. Two of these patients required neck osteotomies with insertion of wedge-shaped autologous tricortical iliac crest bone graft to correct varus malalignment and underwent concurrent stable internal fixation. One of these patients had a coinciding subtalar fusion, and the second went on to develop AVN requiring an ankle fusion. Nevertheless, the investigators also stressed how the restoration of the talus architecture through secondary anatomic reconstruction could produce a favorable outcome. This procedure reestablishes the contact characteristics of the peritalar joints and restricts future arthritic changes, permitting joint preservation or limited hindfoot arthrodesis instead of more advanced salvage procedures.[3]

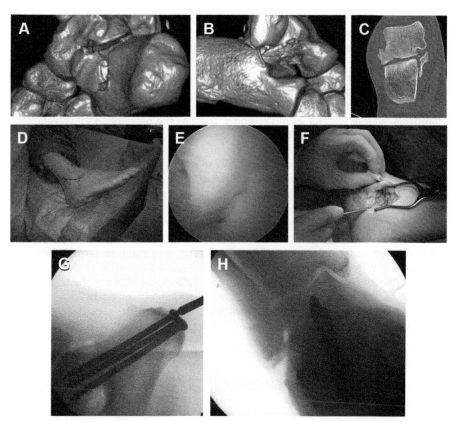

Fig. 3. A 56-year-old male firefighter fell off his mountain cycle, fracturing the sustentaculum tali and lateral talar process. The fracture was treated nonoperatively at a separate hospital and referred to the senior authors' hospital with persisting hindfoot and forefoot varus plus a stiff and painful hindfoot. The patient was unable to work. (*A, B*) A medial view of a 3-dimensional CT reconstruction of the hindfoot demonstrating the sustentaculum tali fracture of the calcaneus and a lateral view showing a lateral talar process fracture. (*C*) A coronal cut through both fractures. (*D*) The patient consented to subtalar arthroscopy, possible osteotomy, and reduction of the fracture fragments or subtalar fusion, dependent on the status of the subtalar joint. The position on the operating table for this procedure is shown. (*E*) A subtalar arthroscopic view confirming extensive cartilage damage to the subtalar joint. (*F*) Removal of the lateral talar fragment to allow reduction and access to the subtalar joint. (*G, H*) Position of the screws for the subtalar fusion. The patient has healed with better hindfoot alignment and is pain-free.

REORIENTATING ARTHRODESIS

In cases of talar malunions and nonunions in which deformity has resulted in joint incongruity and ultimately posttraumatic arthritis, salvage procedures are justified. These procedures include reorientating arthrodesis of the ankle, subtalar, or talonavicular joints (**Fig. 3**).[1,2,4,5] Because the talonavicular joint is rarely affected directly, every effort should be made to preserve it, particularly if both the ankle and subtalar joints are to be fused.[2] A multitude of fixation options exist for these arthrodeses procedures in the wake of posttraumatic arthritis. Standard approaches are used unless the condition of the soft-tissue envelope dictates otherwise. As always, meticulous attention to coronal, sagittal, and axial alignment is required. The principles involved in correcting the deformity include reestablishment of physiologic valgus, lengthening of the medial column, or shortening of the lateral column in conjunction with derotation of the forefoot. Perfect hindfoot alignment is a prerequisite to achieving a stable plantigrade foot.

Where both posttraumatic ankle and subtalar arthritis exist, tibiotalocalcaneal arthrodesis, with or without astragalectomy, remains the only option for salvage.[2,6,9] The results for triple arthrodesis for talar malunions and nonunions are poor.[2,3,9,10]

Although arthrodeses can provide substantial pain relief and a stable plantigrade foot, functional impairment prevails, and the long-term outcome is limited due to the development of degenerative changes in the adjacent joints.[2,3,9,11,12] In this regard, TAA has emerged as a viable alternative to ankle arthrodesis for the operative management of debilitating end-stage posttraumatic arthritis.[32-34] Long-standing concerns with accelerated degeneration of adjacent joints, alterations in gait mechanics, limitations in activity, and the rate of nonunions compelled surgeons to pursue the theoretic advantages offered by TAA. Short-term and medium-term results are encouraging, with an overall failure rate of approximately 10% at 5 years.[32,33] However, caution is warranted in the presence of talar dome AVN or defects, because failure of osseous integration of the talar component may occur due to poor vascularity, and lack of structural support may predispose to subsidence. TAA is particularly useful as a motion-conserving procedure in combination with subtalar and midtarsal fusions.

SUMMARY

Posttraumatic malalignment after talar neck fractures invariably leads to painful functional impairment. Anatomic reduction and definitive, stable osteosynthesis at the primary surgical intervention is preventative. Secondary anatomic reconstruction with joint preservation should be considered in the absence of arthrosis in the peritalar articulations. Reorientating arthrodeses should be entertained where deformity has resulted in joint incongruity and, ultimately, posttraumatic arthritis. TAA may have a role as a motion-conserving procedure in combination with adjacent subtalar and midtarsal fusions.

REFERENCES

1. Rammelt S, Winkler J, Heineck J, et al. Anatomical reconstruction of malunited talus fractures: a prospective study of 10 patients followed for 4 years. Acta Orthop 2005;76(4):588–96.
2. Rammelt S, Winkler J, Grass R, et al. Reconstruction after talar fractures. Foot Ankle Clin 2006;11(1):61–84.
3. Huang PJ, Cheng YM. Delayed surgical treatment for neglected or mal-reduced talar fractures. Int Orthop 2005;29(5):326–9.
4. Fortin PT, Balazsy JE. Talus fractures: evaluation and treatment. J Am Acad Orthop Surg 2001;9(2):114–27.
5. Monroe MT, Manoli A 2nd. Osteotomy for malunion of a talar neck fracture: a case report. Foot Ankle Int 1999;20(3):192–5.
6. Rammelt S, Zwipp H. Talar neck and body fractures. Injury 2009;40(2):120–35.
7. Daniels TR, Smith JW, Ross TI. Varus malalignment of the talar neck. Its effect on the position of the foot and on subtalar motion. J Bone Joint Surg Am 1996;78–A(10):1559–67.
8. Vallier HA, Nork SE, Barie DP, et al. Talar neck fractures: results and outcomes. J Bone Joint Surg Am 2004;86–A(8):1616–24.

9. Calvert E, Younger A, Penner M. Post talus neck fracture reconstruction. Foot Ankle Clin 2007;12(1):137–51.
10. Canale ST, Kelly FB Jr. Fractures of the neck of the talus. J Bone Joint Surg Am 1978;60:143–56.
11. Coester LM, Saltzman CL, Leopold J, et al. Long term results following ankle arthrodesis for post-traumatic arthritis. J Bone Joint Surg Am 2001;83–A:219–28.
12. Kitaoka HB, Patzer GL. Arthrodesis for the treatment of arthrosis of the ankle and osteonecrosis of the talus. J Bone Joint Surg Am 1998;80–A(3):370–9.
13. Sangeorzan BJ, Wagner UA, Harrington RM, et al. Contact characteristics of the subtalar joint: the effect of talar neck misalignment. J Orthop Res 1992;10:544–51.
14. Chan G, Sanders DW, Yuan X, et al. Clinical accuracy of imaging techniques for talar neck malunion. J Orthop Trauma 2008;22(6):415–8.
15. Furlong J, Morrison WB, Carrino JA. Imaging of the talus. Foot Ankle Clin 2004;9(4):685–701.
16. Early JS. Management of fractures of the talus: body and head regions. Foot Ankle Clin 2004;9(4):709–22.
17. Zwipp H, Rammelt S. Post-traumatic deformity correction at the foot. Zentralbl Chir 2003;128(3):219.
18. Ohl X, Harisboure A, Hemery X, et al. Long-term follow-up after surgical treatment of talar fractures: twenty cases with an average follow-up of 7.5 years. Int Orthop 2011;35(1):93–9.
19. Early JS. Talus fracture management. Foot Ankle Clin 2008;13(4):635–57.
20. Ahmad J, Raikin SM. Current concepts review: talar fractures. Foot Ankle Int 2006; 26(6):475–82.
21. Juliano PJ, Dabbah M, Harris TG. Talar neck fractures. Foot Ankle Clin 2004;9(4):723–36.
22. Lindvall E, Haidukewych G, DiPasquale T, et al. Open reduction and stable fixation of isolated, displaced talar neck and body fractures. J Bone Joint Surg Am 2004;86–A(10):2229–34.
23. Archdeacon M, Wilber R. Fractures of the talar neck. Orthop Clin North Am 2002; 33(1):247–62.
24. Daniels TR, Smith JW. Talar neck fractures. Foot Ankle 1993;14:225–34.
25. Grob D, Simpson LA, Weber BG, et al. Operative treatment of displaced talus fractures. Clin Orthop 1985;199:88–96.
26. Higgins TF, Baumgaertner MR. Diagnosis and treatment of fractures of the talus: a comprehensive review of the literature. Foot Ankle Int 1999;20(9):595–605.
27. Saunders DW, Busam M, Hattwick E, et al. Functional outcomes following displaced talar neck fractures. J Orthop Trauma 2004;18(5):265–70.
28. Frawley PA, Hart JA, Young DA. Treatment outcome of major fractures of the talus. Foot Ankle Int 1995;16(6):339–45.
29. Schulze W, Richter J, Russe O, et al. Surgical treatment of talus fractures: a retrospective study of 80 cases followed for 1–15 years. Acta Orthop Scand 2002; 73:344–51.
30. Weinfeld SB. Surgical approaches to the talus. Foot Ankle Clin 2004;9(4):703–8.
31. Fleuriau Chateau PB, Brokaw DS, Jelen BA, et al. Plate fixation of talar neck fractures: preliminary review of a new technique in twenty-three patients J Orthop Trauma 2002;16(4):213–9.
32. Guyer AJ, Richardson G. Current concepts review: total ankle arthroplasty. Foot Ankle Int 2008;29(2):256–64.
33. Gougoulias N, Khanna A, Maffulli N. How successful are current ankle replacement?: a systematic review of the literature. Clin Orthop Relat Res 2010;468(1):199–208.
34. Hintermann B, Valderrabano V. Total ankle replacement. Foot Ankle Clin 2003;8: 375–405.

Total Ankle Replacement in Ankle Arthritis with Varus Talar Deformity: Pathophysiology, Evaluation, and Management Principles

D. Josh Mayich, MD, FRCS(C)[a], Timothy R. Daniels, MD, FRCS(C)[a,b],*

KEYWORDS

- End-stage ankle arthritis • Total ankle replacements
- Varus malalignment of the ankle
- Varus coronal plane deformity of the talus

VMAA is common in end-stage ankle arthritis with varying and poorly described etiologies.[1,2] With a greater understanding of VMAA, it is becoming apparent that its pathology has both hereditary and environmental[3] factors that follow several different pathways, all resulting in a varus coronal plane deformity of the talus. Multiple surgical methods to correct VMAA have been proposed, based primarily on the degree of deformity in the coronal plane.[2,4–7] However, focusing exclusively on the talar coronal plane deformity is an oversimplification of a complex problem.[4,8] The multidimensional nature of VMAA needs to be appreciated by the treating surgeon such that appropriate interventions can be planned in advance of the surgery.[9–11] The purpose of this article is to describe the current understanding of the varus coronal plane deformity of the talus and to summarize the senior author's surgical approach to managing VMAA during TAR.

PATHOANATOMY AND CLASSIFICATION

Recent research into the functional role of the medial peritalar structures, ankle joint biomechanics, and VMAA have advanced our understanding of end-stage ankle joint

The authors have nothing to disclose.
[a] St. Michael's Hospital, 800-55 Queen Street East, Toronto, ON, Canada M5C 1R6
[b] Foot & Ankle Program, University of Toronto, Toronto, ON, Canada
* Corresponding author. St. Michael's Hospital, 800-55 Queen Street East, Toronto, ON, Canada M5C 1R6.
E-mail address: DanielsT@smh.ca

arthritis.[9,10,12–17] This has led to the development of deformity- and treatment-based classification systems or definitions of VMAA to help with preoperative and intraoperative decision making.[5,8,18] These classification systems focus almost entirely on a single orthoganal plane of deformity and do not necessarily address the multiplanar nature of VMAA, particularly the rotational deformities in the transverse plane. A thorough evaluation of the entire lower extremity, both clinically and radiographically, is necessary to develop an appropriate individualized surgical plan.[3,19,20]

Clinical Evaluation

The clinical history must rule out neurologic causes such as hereditary sensory motor neuropathies, tethered spinal cord, peripheral nerve injury, clubfoot, or subclinical nonprogressive neurologic abnormalities such as mild cerebral palsy. A history of these etiologies may be subtle and can be a contraindication for TAR. Often, patients with a history of progressive hindfoot varus have functioned at a high level for many years despite radiographic evidence of advanced ankle arthritis and hindfoot deformity. It is not uncommon for an event such as ruptured peroneus longus and/or brevis tendons or other minor traumatic occurrences to precipitate rapid radiographic and clinical deterioration.

A complete evaluation of the entire lower extremity is an important first step in the physical examination. Special attention should be paid to the orientation of the knee and tibia: In the presence of a significant genu varus, there may be knee arthritis as well as hindfoot varus. This is not uncommon in patients over 60 years of age. In these clinical scenarios, a more proximal tibial osteotomy or knee arthroplasty may be required before addressing the ankle and hindfoot pathology (**Fig. 1**). Observation of gait is essential, with particular focus on (i) the varus thrust of the knee during mid-stance, (ii) knee contractures, (iii) the pattern of heel–progression, (iv) a rigid or increased hindfoot varus during stance phase, and (v) ruling out any clinical evidence of weak dorsiflexion—namely, high stepping drop foot gait.

As described by Ryssman and Myerson,[20] a focused examination of the ankle includes the degree and location of deformity, range of motion (ROM) and stability of the peritalar joints. Documentation of any contributing deformities, such as midfoot cavus and noting the apex below the level of the ankle, are important.[21] Particular attention is directed to the arc of peritalar motion. If the hindfoot cannot be everted past the neutral position, this may indicate substantial medial contractures that need to be addressed at the time of surgery. Patients with this clinical finding often have significant transverse plane rotational deformities that occur at multiple joints including the ankle, subtalar, Chopart and midtarsal joints.

Weak eversion suggests a rupture of one or both of the peroneal tendons. In these cases, it is important to perform a posterior tibial tendon (PTT) to peroneus brevis and/or peroneus longus to peroneus brevis transfer with lateral ankle ligament reconstruction. Attention should be paid to the neurologic examination, including the major domains of nerve function and vascular supply to the foot. Any documented or suspected abnormal findings need further investigation.

Radiographic Evaluation

Radiographic evaluation is ultimately driven by the findings on clinical evaluation. Findings outside of the ankle and foot should be documented and localized using appropriate imaging: Specifically, frontal plane malalignment of the lower extremity using a teleoroentgenogram (in cases of leg length discrepancy, with or without correction of the leg length deficit) or, for a more complex deformity, a computed tomography scanogram in addition to plain radiographs.

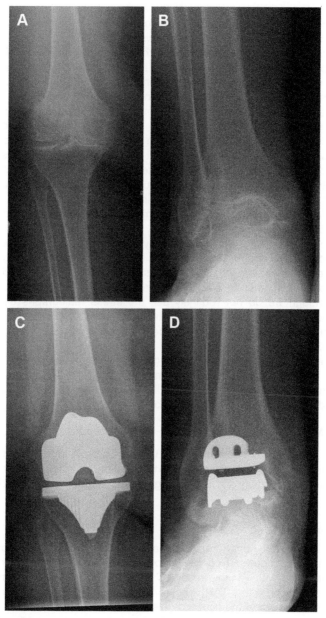

Fig. 1. (*A*) Standing anteroposterior (AP) of the knee identifying medial compartment osteoarthritis with varus deformity. (*B*) Standing AP of the ankle on the same patient with a congruent varus ankle deformity. (*C*) Standing AP of the Knee after a total knee arthroplasty with correction of varus deformity. (*D*) Standing AP of the ankle on the same patient after total ankle arthroplasty with correction of the varus deformity.

Standard radiographic examination of the ankle includes orthogonal, full-length, weight-bearing tibial radiographs, and anteroposterior and lateral hindfoot views. Maximal dorsiflexion and plantar-flexion views of the ankle as well as lateral and oblique views of the foot are optional. On the anteroposterior view of the ankle, attention is paid to the degree of coronal talar plane deformity, orientation of the tibial plafond (ie, congruent vs incongruent deformity), evidence of previous fractures, and the orientation and condition of the medial malleolus. Typically, congruent varus deformities are stiffer and more difficult to correct than incongruent deformities (**Fig. 2**). In approximately 25% of cases, the medial malleolus can be flared in a medial direction, creating a void in the anteromedial aspect of the ankle mortise (**Figs. 3**A and **4**A). On the lateral weight-bearing ankle view, the position of the talus is noted as well as the integrity of the anterior aspect of the tibial plafond. In our experience, the more anterior the talus is subluxed, the greater the internal rotational deformity of the talus and the greater likelihood of the presence of substantial anterolateral impinging osteophytes, a larger medial talar osteophyte, and deficiency of the anterior tibial plafond (**Fig. 5**).

We also routinely obtain the modified Cobey view of the hindfoot, as described by Saltzman and el-Khoury[22] and substantiated clinically by Frigg and colleagues.[23] This view is particularly useful in postoperative assessment of hindfoot position and it helps to determine whether ancillary procedures such as calcaneal osteotomies are required. Although we do not routinely use the stress radiographs described by Ryssman and Myerson[20] in the preoperative phase, this is a standard procedure performed in the operating room before the start of the operation with the patient anesthetized.

In cases of (a) questionable bone stock, (b) significant rotational malalignment, or (c) adjacent joint disease, computed tomography of the ankle and foot using radiation-minimizing protocols is typically utilized (magnetic resonance imaging of the foot and ankle in the setting of coronal deformity is rarely utilized).

OPERATIVE MANAGEMENT

Once formal evaluation of the patient and VMAA has been performed, the treating surgeon should understand which lower extremity abnormalities are contributing to the varus hindfoot deformity and which surgical interventions are required to correct them.

Nonarthroplasty

The 2 main options for nonarthroplasty management of VMAA are supramalleolar osteotomy and arthrodesis. Recently, supramalleolar osteotomies have received increasing attention with variable results.[15,24,25] A tibial–fibular osteotomy may be required in association with a TAR[11]; however, discussion of its role in management of ankle arthritis is beyond the scope of this article.

Arthroplasty/Replacement

The decision to proceed with TAR in a patient with significant VMAA is attained only after careful counseling and thorough evaluation.[3,5,10,13,18,19,26] The goals of TAR in VMAA are to (1) place all components perpendicular to the plumb line of the body, such that when the patient stands up, the components are parallel to the floor in all planes, (2) achieve a balanced, stable, congruent ankle joint with plantigrade alignment of the hindfoot and forefoot; and (3) restore as much ankle ROM as possible.[3,18,27] If these criteria cannot be met, a fusion should be performed.[27,28]

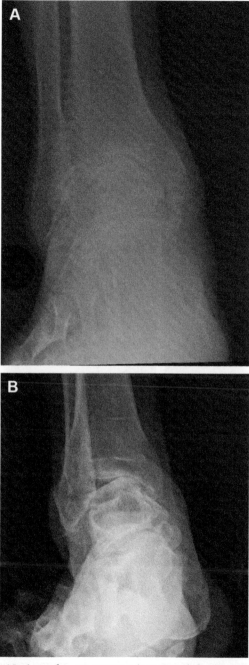

Fig. 2. (*A*) Standing AP view of a congruent talar varus deformity. Note that the talus is incased by osteophytes and the tibial plafonde has gradually molded to the shape of the varus oriented talus. (*B*) Standing AP of an incongruent talar varus deformity. Note that the talus and tibial plafonde have maintained their original shape.

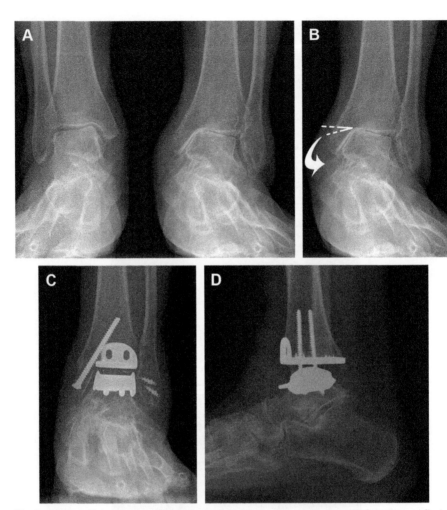

Fig. 3. (*A*) Standing anteroposterior view of a patient with a talar varus deformity and flaring of the medial malleolus. Note the increased volume of the ankle mortise with a gap laterally as the talus has rotated in an internal and medial direction. (*B*) Location of opening wedge medial malleolar osteotomy with arrow indicating the external rotation required to correct the deformity. (*C*) Ankle mortise normalized with use of a medial based opening wedge malleolar osteotomy. Note that the medial malloelus needs to be closed and rotated externally to re-orientate it back to its normal anatomic position. (*D*) Lateral view after medial malleolar osteotomy.

Once the patient is fully anesthetized, the ankle is physically examined. A valgus and eversion stress determines the flexibility of the hindfoot: The more rigid the deformity, the greater the number of ancillary procedures required to correct the deformity. Attention is paid to the ability to evert the foot past neutral; if this is not possible, a significant medial release is required. Preoperative planning should have determined whether a tibial osteotomy (proximal or distal) and/or total knee replacement is necessary (it is not uncommon for these 2 procedures to be performed in 1 surgical setting at our institution).

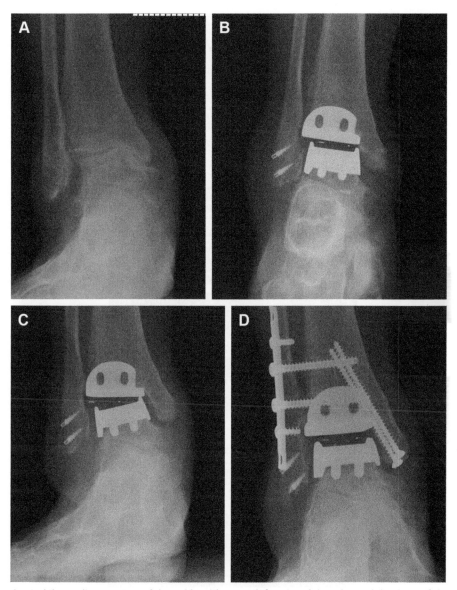

Fig. 4. (*A*) Standing AP view of the ankle with varus deformity of the talus and dysplasia of the medial malleolus. (*B*) Four weeks postoperative AP view before patient begins to bear weight. (*C*) Three-month postoperative, weight-bearing AP view demonstrating the recurrent varus deformity. The talus has internally rotated and fallen into the defect created by the dysplasia of the medial malleolus. (*D*) One-year postoperative, weight bearing AP view after medial malleolar biplanar opening wedge/external rotation osteotomy and stabilization of syndesmosis.

Approach and initial release
The standard anterior approach is employed.[13,18,27] Once the ankle is adequately exposed, osteophytes—typically located on the anterolateral plafond (hypertrophied tubercle of Chaput), the lateral gutter (talus and fibula), and the anteromedial surfaces

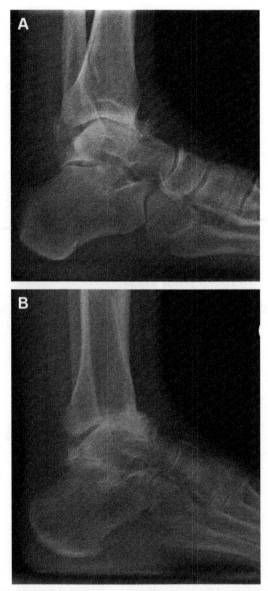

Fig. 5. (*A*) Standing lateral radiograph demonstrating some anterior translation of the talus. The abnormal appearance of the talus is created by the varus and internal rotation position of the talus, creating an oblique rather than direct lateral of the talus. (*B*) Standing lateral radiograph of a patient with increased anterior translation. Note the deficiency of the anterior tibial plafonde combined with subtalar joint arthritis. When performing the tibial cut, the deficiency of bone anteriorly needs to be taken into consideration such that excessive tibial bone resection does not result.

of the talus and the anterior aspect of the medial malleolus—are thoroughly debrided. There is often a shelf-osteophyte extending off of the medial aspect of the talar body and neck that requires extensive debridement (**Fig. 5**A). At this point, the correctability of the talus is evaluated. The surgeon applies a valgus stress to the hindfoot: (a) If the talar varus corrects, a posterior and external rotation force is applied at the ankle, and the talus should externally rotate and reduce into the ankle mortise; (b) if the talus does not correct, then a deltoid/medial release and further debridement of the lateral ankle joint is required.[13,18,27] This includes a release of the posterior portion of the deep deltoid ligament as well as a release of the posterior lateral aspect of the ankle, which includes debridement of the often hypertrophied calcaneofibular and posterior syndesmotic ligaments.[18,27]

If the talar reduction is still difficult and the foot does not evert past neutral, then—through separate incisions—a plantar fascia release, lengthening of the PTT and release of the talonavicular capsule are performed. Once the medial release is completed to the surgeon's satisfaction, then the aforementioned reduction technique is performed once more. At this time, if deemed necessary, the PTT is prepared for transfer to the peroneus brevis tendon. A posteromedial incision is made approximately 5 cm above the medial malleolus and the PTT is delivered proximally; then, the PTT is transferred along the back of the tibia and fibula by safe standard techniques to the lateral aspect of the ankle into the peroneal tendon sheath. The final sutures attaching the PTT to the peroneus brevis tendon are performed after the total ankle components are in place, followed by a lateral ligament repair (the senior author has a low threshold for performing a PTT transfer given the powerful effect it has on maintaining correction of the hindfoot varus). As supported by Ryssman and Myerson,[20] Doets and co-workers[29] describe and advocate a sliding medial malleolar osteotomy in place and/or in association with a medial release (the authors of this chapter have no experience with this technique).

Coetzee[18] raised valid concerns about the neurovascular structures during medial and lateral ligament release. According to Daniels and associates,[27] however, the neurovascular structures are not at risk as long as the periosteal elevator is kept directly on bone and controlled movements are used. A final direct view of the ankle is then secured utilizing laminar spreaders, and any remaining osteophytes are resected. The laminar spreaders also tension the tissue. This is carried out in both plantarflexion and dorsiflexion to (1) ensure that there is no gross asymmetry after releases and (2) allow for further evaluation of the progress made in balancing the ankle.

If complete correction of the coronal deformity is not obtainable, then (as previously highlighted by Daniels and colleagues,[27] and Ryssman and Myerson[20]) a separate anterolateral incision is made over the distal fibula; this incision may have already been made if a PTT transfer has been deemed necessary. The orientation and length of the lateral incision are customized to what lateral work is required. The remnant of the anterior tibiofibular ligament and the ankle joint capsule are dissected off the fibula. Any remaining or previously unrecognized anterior–inferior fibular and lateral talar body osteophytes are removed. Care is taken not to violate the sinus tarsi. The crucial deltoid branches and anterior blood supply to the talus are likely sacrificed in previous stages of the operation.[6,15] Furthermore, the effect of the pathologic process of VMAA and its resultant deformity on the blood supply of the talus is not defined.[6,15]

Sagittal balancing

After the attempted balancing, ankle ROM is assessed for any hinging. Most commonly, this occurs in ankles with severe initial deformity and in those with lateral laxity.[3] Restoring the tibiotalar ratio or the anteroposterior offset ratio and sagittal balance to this multiplanar deformity is the goal of the surgery—this predicates the success of the TAR.[8,30] By contrast, any residual sagittal imbalance could lead to abnormal biomechanical function of TAR and premature failure.[30] The preoperative goal of restoring ROM is addressed here as well. Before proceeding with any bone cuts, we arbitrarily use 45° as a reference point.

Tibia bone preparation

Attention is then turned to the tibia. In the condition of VMAA, dysplasia of the medial malleolus is well described.[20,31] Even in the mild cases, orientation of the morphology of the medial malleolus must be carefully considered. The tibial cutting guide is aligned with the medial aspect of the ankle mortise (rather than the medial malleolus) when significant dysplasia is present (see **Figs. 3**A and **4**A).

Bone cuts are performed first on the tibial side. All tibial cuts are made to include any medial plafond defects so as to maximize contact of the tibial prosthesis on the bone.[32] The external rotational deformity of the ankle mortise that often accompanies VMAA is crucial to recognize before making any cuts. This is done by distracting the talus with laminar spreaders or similar devices and directly visualizing the orientation of the malleoli. This allows the rotation of the tibial cutting guide to be matched to the native rotation of the ankle mortise.

Talar bone preparation

After the tibial cut, the talus is addressed. The importance of obtaining/maintaining a concentric reduction of the talus at this point cannot be overemphasized. After the talar cuts and implantation of the trial components, ROM and the concentric nature of the medial–lateral and sagittal balancing are assessed. If imbalance is noted, then evaluation of the bone cuts and implant location with fluoroscopy can be undertaken, followed by any necessary corrections. If there is global tightness, additional tibial resection can be employed; 2-mm increments are suggested to preserve as much tibial bone stock as possible.[32] A final attempt at any soft tissue balancing, gutter debridement, and osteophyte resection should be undertaken.

Medial malleolar osteotomy

Once the ankle components are in place, the orientation of the medial malleolus and the translational stability of the talus are assessed. In cases where there is significant dysplasia or medial orientation of the medial malleolus, a medial-based opening wedge osteotomy is performed (**Fig. 3**B). The medial malleolus is osteotomized transversely, at the level of the tibial component, followed by a biplanar repositioning of the malleolus, which involves rotating it externally and opening it medially. This closes the anterolateral gap and stabilizes the talar component. If this is not performed, the talus can quickly fall into varus when the patient begins to bear weight (**Fig. 4**).

Addressing the foot deformity

After the ankle joint replacement is stable and necessary tendon transfers completed, our final focus shifts to evaluation of the foot. Attention is paid to evaluating the Achilles tendon, heel alignment, hindfoot ROM, and any accompanying forefoot deformity—most commonly, a plantarflexed first ray. The senior author seldom performs a calcaneal osteotomy or tendoachilles lengthening because these procedures are not required if proper attention has been paid to appropriate soft tissue release and rebalancing.

In summary, the most common ancillary procedures performed surrounding TAR for VMAA consist of (i) plantar fascia release, (ii) lengthening and/or transfer of the PTT, (iii) medial malleolar osteotomy, (iv) dorsiflexion osteotomy of the first metatarsal, and (v) lateral ligament reconstruction.

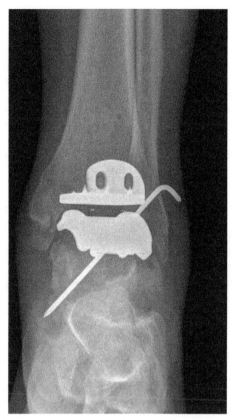

Fig. 6. A large K-wire is passed from the fibula into the talus, below the talar component, to stabilize the ankle in both the coronal and sagittal planes while the soft tissues heal. The K-wire is removed at 4 weeks postoperatively.

Persistent talar varus instability

Aside from attempting TAR in the presence of VMAA, perhaps the most difficult decision to make is converting an ankle prepared for a TAR to a fusion based on an intraoperative inability to balance the ankle or achieve a stable articulating TAR. If, after having followed the strict surgical goals outlined in the beginning of this section, the talar component is correctable but falls into varus as the corrective forces are removed, then medial and/or lateral K-wires are inserted with the ankle reduced and in neutral position. The K-wires are buried subcutaneously and removed at 4 to 5 weeks (**Fig. 6**). If the ankle simply cannot be balanced, then the ankle is converted to a fusion (the senior author has had 6 such cases to date). The anticipated loss of height that occurred did not seem to be an issue beyond shoe modifications. Good results have been reported at midterm follow up—a contrast with the predictably poor results reported on patients with a poorly balanced (or "edge-loading") TAR.[5,28] As in all cases for TAR with VMAA, patients are counseled and prepared preoperatively that they may, in fact, wake from the anesthesia with their ankle joint fused rather than replaced. In time, any initial disappointment wanes as the patient begins to enjoy the reliably good outcomes from a fusion in the context of VMAA.[13]

SUMMARY

Varus malalignment of the ankle may be a misleading term. The isolated frontal plane deformity has been shown to be multiplanar in nature. Identifying this dominant feature of the condition and applying appropriate surgical principles to allow for complete correction of the deformity are critical to a successful outcome. The following 3 factors are key to an optimal surgical outcome from TAR with VMAA: (1) Obtaining a congruent ankle with sufficient ROM is a important before implantation of the arthroplasty prosthesis; (2) not all ankles are correctable; and (3) recognition both preoperatively and intraoperatively that a conversion of TAR to a fusion is sometimes the best course of action to achieve best results or patient satisfaction.

REFERENCES

1. Tochigi Y, Takahashi K, Yamagata M, et al. Influence of the interosseous talocalcaneal ligament injury on stability of the ankle-subtalar joint complex—a cadaveric experimental study. Foot Ankle Int 2000;21:486–91.
2. Valderrabano V, Horisberger M, Russell I, et al. Etiology of ankle osteoarthritis. Clin Orthop Relat Res 2009;467:1800–6.
3. Hennessy MS, Molloy AP, Wood EV. Management of the varus arthritic ankle. Foot Ankle Clin North Am 2008;13:417–42.
4. Doets HC, Brand R, Nelissen RGHH. Total ankle arthroplasty in inflammatory joint disease with use of two mobile-bearing designs. J Bone Joint Surg Am 2006;88-A: 1272–84.
5. Haskell A, Mann RA. Ankle arthroplasty with pre-operative coronal plane deformity: short term results. Clin Orthop Relat Res 2004;424:98–103.
6. Kelikian AS, editor. Sarrafian's anatomy of the foot and ankle. Descriptive, topographic, functional. 3rd edition. Philadelphia: Wolters Kluwer/Lippincott Williams & Wilkins; 2011.
7. Wood PL, Prem H, Sutton C. Total ankle replacement: medium-term results in 200 Scandinavian total ankle replacements. J Bone Joint Surg Br 2008;90:605–9.
8. Wood PLR, Sutton C, Mishra V, et al. A randomized, controlled trial of two mobile-bearing total ankle replacements. J Bone Joint Surg [Br] 2009;91-B:69–74.
9. Daniels TR, Thomas R. Etiology and biomechanics of ankle arthritis. Foot Ankle Clin North Am 2008;13:341–52.
10. Knupp M, Stufkens SAS, van Bergen CJ, et al. Effect of supramalleolar varus and valgus deformities on the tibiotalar joint: a cadaveric study. Foot Ankle Int 2011;32: 609–15.
11. Smith R, Wood PLR. Arthrodesis of the ankle in the presence of a large deformity in the coronal plane. J Bone Joint Surg [Br] 2007;89-B:615–9.
12. Ellis SJ, Williams BR, Wagshul AD, et al. Deltoid ligament reconstruction with peroneus longus autograft in flatfoot deformity. Foot Ankle Int 2010;31781–8.
13. Greissberg J, Hansen ST, DiGiovanni C. Alignment and technique in total ankle arthroplasty. Oper Tech Orthop 2004;14:21–30.
14. Lee WC, Moon JS, Lee HS, et al. Alignment of ankle and hindfoot in early stage ankle osteoarthritis. Foot Ankle Int 2011;32:693–9.
15. Prasarn ML, Miller AN, Dyke JP, et al. Arterial anatomy of the talus: a cadaver and gadolinium-enhanced MRI study. Foot Ankle Int 2010;31:987–93.
16. Stufkens SA, van Bergen CJ, Blankevoort L, et al. The role of the fibula in varus and valgus deformity of the tibia: A Biomechanical study. J Bone Joint Surg [Br] 2011;93-B:1232–9.

17. Tochigi Y, Rudert MJ, Saltzman CL, et al. Contribution of articular surface geometry to ankle stabilization. J Bone Joint Surg Am 2006;88-A:2704–13.
18. Coetzee JC. Management of the varus or valgus ankle deformity with ankle replacement. Foot Ankle Clin North Am 2008;13:509–20.
19. LaClair SM. Reconstruction of the varus ankle from soft-tissue procedures with osteotomy through arthrodesis. Foot Ankle Clin North Am 2007;12:153–76.
20. Ryssman D, Myerson MS. Surgical strategies: the management of varus ankle deformity with joint replacement. Foot Ankle Int 2011;32:217–24.
21. Davis HW, Mann RA. Principles of the physical examination of the foot and ankle. In: Coughlin MJ, Mann RA, Saltzman CL, editors. Surgery of the foot and ankle. 8th edition. Philadelphia: Mosby Elsevier; 2009.
22. Saltzman CL, el-Khoury GY. The hindfoot alignment view. Foot Ankle Int 1995;16: 572–6.
23. Frigg A, Nigg B, Hinz L, et al. Clinical relevance of hindfoot alignment view in total ankle replacement. Foot Ankle Int 2010;31:871–9.
24. Banthien RA, Myerson MS. Supramalleolar osteotomy for ankle deformity and arthritis. Foot Ankle Clin North Am 2004;9:475–87.
25. Lee W-C, Moon J-S, Lee K, et al. Indications for supramalleolar osteotomy in patients with ankle osteoarthritis and varus deformity. J Bone Joint Surg Am 2011;93-A: 1243–8.
26. Kim BS, Choi WJ, Kim YS, et al. Total ankle replacement in moderate to severe varus deformity of the ankle. J Bone Joint Surg [Br] 2009;91-B:1183–90.
27. Daniels TR, Cadden AR, Lim KK. Correction of varus total deformities in ankle joint replacement. Oper Tech Orthop 2008;18:282–6.
28. Hobson SA, Karantana A, Dhar S. Total ankle replacement in patients with significant pre-operative deformity of the hindfoot. J Bone Joint Surg [Br] 2009;91-B:481–6.
29. Doets HC, van der Plaat LW, Klein J-P. Medial malleolar osteotomy for the correction of varus deformity during total ankle arthroplasty: results in 15 ankles. Foot Ankle Int 2008;29:171–7.
30. Barg A, Elsner A, Anderson AE, et al. The effect of three-component total ankle replacement malalignment on clinical outcome: pain relief and functional outcome in 317 consecutive patients. J Bone Joint Surg Am 2011;93:1969–78.
31. Merian M, Glisson RR, Nunley JA. Ligament balancing for total ankle arthroplasty: an in vitro evaluation of the elongation of the hind- and mid-foot ligaments. Foot Ankle Int 2011;32:457.
32. Hintermann B. Total ankle arthroplasty. Historical overview, current concepts and future perspectives. Vienna (Austria): Springer-Verlag; 2005.

Index

Note: Page numbers of article titles are in **boldface** type.

Foot Ankle Clin N Am 17 (2012) 141–168
doi:10.1016/S1083-7515(12)00009-5
1083-7515/12/$ – see front matter © 2012 Elsevier Inc. All rights reserved.

Moving?

Make sure your subscription moves with you!

To notify us of your new address, find your **Clinics Account Number** (located on your mailing label above your name), and contact customer service at:

Email: journalscustomerservice-usa@elsevier.com

800-654-2452 (subscribers in the U.S. & Canada)
314-447-8871 (subscribers outside of the U.S. & Canada)

Fax number: 314-447-8029

Elsevier Health Sciences Division
Subscription Customer Service
3251 Riverport Lane
Maryland Heights, MO 63043

*To ensure uninterrupted delivery of your subscription, please notify us at least 4 weeks in advance of move.

Printed and bound by CPI Group (UK) Ltd, Croydon, CR0 4YY

03/10/2024

01040455-0015